Antonia has been a teacher for 12 years and is currently Senior Leader Director of English. She is married to Tony and has two daughters, Liliana and Alba. When not teaching or spending time with her family, her hobbies include working behind the scenes with a local theatre company; sports including skiing, ballet and swimming; and curling up with a good book.

For my mum, Dee

# Antonia Chapman-Jones

# I STAND AMAZED...

AUSTIN MACAULEY PUBLISHERS™

LONDON • CAMBRIDGE • NEW YORK • SHARJAH

A CIP catalogue record for this title is available from the British Library.

ISBN 9781528925419 (Paperback)
ISBN 9781528925426 (Kindle e-book)
ISBN 9781528964296 (ePub e-book)

www.austinmacauley.com

First Published (2019)
Austin Macauley Publishers Ltd
25 Canada Square
Canary Wharf
London
E14 5LQ

I would like to start by thanking my dad, Ian, for all his help and support, not just with this book but with any problem I have had over the years.

I am indebted to my wonderful husband, Tony. He's my rock and without his patience and love (and tough words at times), this would not have been a possibility.

Thank you to my wonderful girls who gave me my reason for getting up on a morning.

And finally, my army of angels – too many to name but all of whom I hold close in my heart. Without you, I would not be the person I am today – you know who you are.

One family's battle against Acute Myeloid Leukaemia.

# Hello World

Leukaemia is a deadly and devastating disease. It has touched my family. Here's our journey for all to share.

# The Worst News

This is possibly the hardest message I have ever had to write so please bear with me. Mum has an aggressive form of leukaemia. She starts chemo on Thursday. She will be in hospital for at least a month, will lose her hair and has a huge battle on her hands. However, they are starting very aggressive treatment and have given an 80% prognosis of remission. As you can imagine, we will not take this lying down and will fight it every step of the way.

xxx

# The Story so Far...

So, my mum has been diagnosed with Acute Myeloid Leukaemia. She has gone from being the picture of health and happiness to being extremely ill in a matter of days. At times what I write is very emotional and if anything I write upsets people, then I apologise in advance; this is such a difficult thing to go through and sometimes being polite is just too hard. The truth is that she is gravely ill and has a long hard battle ahead of her. She's the strongest woman I know and for that reason I believe that if anyone can beat this, it is my mum. I wish I could fight this for her but unfortunately the world is unfair. She is amazing, she is special and she is loved. She is my mum and I love her and I will support her every step of the way.

xxx

# Dark Days Despite the Sun

Just wanted to let you know that Mum started chemotherapy today. It was not pleasant and has knocked all the energy out of her. She is feeling very tired and has no energy left at all. She is still in pain from Tuesday's bone marrow aspiration and the insertion of a Hickman line yesterday. The bone marrow aspiration is nasty – basically they drill into your hip and put a huge needle in to draw bone marrow out. It was done under local anaesthetic so wasn't too bad at first but once the anaesthetic wore off, it was incredibly painful for her. She was in pain if she lay on her back as it put pressure on her right hip (the site of the aspiration.) Unfortunately, the following day she had a Hickman line inserted. This is on the left side of her chest and in layman terms it's a tube through which she will receive all medication. It is a semi-permanent tube which means that it will stay in for quite some time. The reason for the line is that it will stop her veins from hardening then crumbling – she will have so many different drips each day that the best course is just to have one site for all medications to go in through. The line doesn't hurt particularly but it does hang down from her chest which is uncomfortable. This meant that she couldn't get comfortable on her right side (bone marrow aspiration site), on her left side (Hickman line) or her back (bone marrow aspiration site). Her front wasn't an option as it would mean lying on the Hickman line (PAINFUL!). The only time I saw her comfortable was sitting up in a chair, resting her head on her arms on the table in front of her. She is also starting to struggle to breathe so is hooked up to oxygen 22 hours out of 24.

She is not really up for visitors yet as she keeps falling asleep mid-sentence. Over the next few weeks she will receive two types of chemo – one twice a day, every day, and the other once every two days. It was the latter type she had today and that is the one that is going to have the biggest impact; both on the leukaemia and on her in general. She is still bruising and today developed two whopping black eyes. She continues to be as beautiful as ever. Please continue praying for her – she needs all our love and support. Thank you for all your support so far – I cannot express how much it means to us all. I will continue these updates (Mum has ordered it – who am I to argue?!) but if you find it at all distressing, then please let me know.

xxx

# The Chemotherapy Begins

Today Mum was more alert. She had chemo yesterday and it knocked her out and this morning she was very tired. She has had a temperature for the past few days and today they gave her some antibiotics and paracetamol in order to break the fever. When her temp came down, she was given a blood transfusion which started to bring her temperature down.

There was good news when we were told that her white blood cell count has gone down – a massive positive. Also, she managed to eat a full dinner today – given the state of hospital food this is a huge achievement in itself, but it means that she is feeling better as in the last few days her appetite had completely vanished. She was more alert today than she has been which is also good but she has 'big' chemo again tomorrow which will mean she would be exhausted again. We must take every day as it comes and celebrate small achievements – we appreciate your support in doing so. Thank you for your prayers and good wishes.

Much love,
Ant

xxx

# What's Going On?

Mum went on holiday – a med cruise followed by a week in the sun – with my dad, my aunt and my uncle. They had an amazing time and came back the picture of health, with tans to die for and stories galore. Two weeks later, she was in the hospital.

I'd never heard of 'Acute Myeloid Leukaemia' before three weeks ago. I'd hear the term 'Leukaemia' and knew that it was some type of cancer that affected the blood; I even knew it was to do with your bone marrow producing too many white blood cells and those blood cells thinking healthy bits of your blood were viruses and attacking them. I thought I was so clever.

But what I didn't know – and I'm not sure how many people would unless they had a reason to know – was that there are different types of Leukaemia. I thought it was something that took years to develop and grew gradually and in some ways I was right. Apparently, *Chronic* Myeloid Leukaemia is a bit like that. But *Acute* Myeloid Leukaemia is different. So in order to spread the word – and awareness – I thought I'd tell you Mum's story and then a little bit about what Mum, Dad and I have learned in the past few weeks.

One Thursday my mum woke up feeling a bit under the weather. She's had a check-up (blood etc.) the week before as she is in remission from bowel cancer. They'd come back clear so she didn't worry too much. A bit of summer flu, we thought. She went to bed early and felt a little better the next morning. So much better that she went to her grandson's sports day (and probably shouted louder than any other spectator!).

On Saturday morning she went to the church to help out with the annual gardening drive. She tore down armfuls of ivy, cleared pathways, dead headed plants and was ruthless when it came to pruning. Whilst bending over to gather another armful of ivy, her top rode up slightly, allowing my dad to glimpse a whopping bruise on her back and hip. It was navy blue and huge. Dad asked what she'd done to get it but she knew she hadn't bashed into anything. Alarm bells started ringing faintly.

That evening, she decided to cancel the prearranged concert and headed for the walk-in clinic. The doctors there said they thought it was something to do with her platelets and that her best bet was to go to her doctor on Monday morning and have a blood test. The bells grew slightly louder.

On Sunday she was tired – very tired – but managed to go to church and sing in the choir, eat cake and have a gossip after the service. However, she went to bed very early and slept like a log.

Early Monday morning she woke up to discover her mouth full of excruciating blood blisters. So painful she couldn't eat or drink. Dad drove her to the doctor's where blood was taken, marked 'urgent' and a follow-up appointment made for the next day. The follow-up appointment was not kept because by then Mum was already in North Tees Hospital. At six thirty on Monday night, she received a phone call from NTH saying there was a bed waiting for her on ward 38 (Haematology) and that she needed to get there ASAP.

By the same time on Tuesday, a specialist had delivered the devastating news that she had Acute Myeloid Leukaemia. A treatment plan was outlined; two types of chemotherapy, one delivered twice a day every day, and one 'big' chemo delivered once a day every other day. Also, she would need IV fluids, antibiotics and various other medications. And she would get very sick; very quickly.

And she did.

She got very sick. So sick that she couldn't stay awake through a sentence. So sick that she needed to be on oxygen

24/7. So sick that she nearly died. And it all happened within a week.

Because that's what happens with Acute Myeloid Leukaemia. Everything in your blood and bone marrow can be working perfectly, then one day it decides to stop playing fair. The bone marrow starts producing more and more and more white blood cells – immature white blood cells – which flood the bone marrow and prevent your blood from clotting. In one day Mum's white cells nearly doubled, going from 80 to 150. A healthy person would have had 20. So the chemotherapy is designed to strip your bone marrow of everything and hopefully start it producing the right levels. Which it is doing. After the first chemo session, her white cell count had come down. But that in turn means that she is more susceptible to infection. For every up there is a down.

So there you go. That's how quickly it can happen. And, without wanting to sound like the awful radio adverts who bang on about all the things that could be wrong with you if you so much as sneeze, this is my plea. That if you feel ill, you call a doctor. It might be nothing, it might be something. But bad things can happen so quickly that isn't it better to get it checked out? Just to be sure.

xxx

# Violet Beauregard Eat Your Heart Out

Hi all,

Yesterday morning Mum was up and went into the garden for a bit of fresh air. It left her completely exhausted but at least she got out of her hospital room and saw a bit of sun. She has been told that she has to have fewer visitors as she is extremely tired and she needs to conserve her energy in order to better fight.

This morning she managed to get into the garden again. She loved it and even snuck a piece of lavender back into her room (if the nurses find it, she'll be for it as she is categorically not allowed to have flowers in her room due to the risk of infection!). She was taken for an x-ray earlier on because she is very breathless and they are a little concerned – this is not a usual side effect and they do not know what is causing it.

Hopefully, we'll know more tomorrow. She has also started to resemble Violet Beauregarde (a la *Charlie and the Chocolate Factory*.) and is swelling up. She even has the purple skin to complete the look! :) The swelling is completely normal and caused by water retention due to the chemo, but this does not make her feel any better. In her words, she is 'monstrous' and although I completely disagree, I have to admit that she looks uncomfortable and in pain. It is so hard to watch because it makes us (Dad and me) feel completely impotent. We can do nothing to ease what she is going through yet we sit by her bedside every day and watch her get worse.

If anything is monstrous, it is this. No one should have to watch someone they love go through this – it is cruel. And no one should have to have people watch them go through it. There is little dignity in this disease. Your instinct is always to protect those you love; to help them fight injustice and seek resolution. The injustice is plain to see but we cannot help. For all our words of support and encouragement and promises to 'help her fight', we are all aware of the hollow ring to the words. We cannot help her fight. We can only hold her hand and wipe away her (very) occasional tears and our (much more frequent) ones; so that is what we continue to do.

She had another 'big' chemo today and so we expect her to be more tired tomorrow. The rhythm is starting to emerge. We spent this evening laughing, giggling and gossiping. It was lovely. Long may these evenings continue.

xxx

# X-Tra, X-Tra, the X-Ray Results Are In

Results are back from the x-ray. Mum has fluid on both her lungs. There are a few possible reasons for this.

1) They have a policy of filling people with fluid when they go to hospital to ensure they do not dehydrate which would affect the chemo/medication they will receive. The fluid in her lungs could be a result of this and the fact that she is not moving very much – the fluid pools at the bottom of her lungs and in her legs (which are incredibly swollen still).
2) The fluid is a result of an infection.
3) The fluid is pus (lovely) and could become a serious complication.

They will not know which it is yet so are going to wait and see how she gets on. In order to be 100% sure, they will have to insert a needle into the fluid and extract some, then test it to see if there is infection present. At the moment, they are not going to do this as it is a painful procedure which is unnecessary at this stage. We are keeping everything crossed that it is the first reason and not the other two. There will be enough painful procedures in the future without her undergoing ones just for the sake of it.

Mum went into the garden this morning and felt the sun on her skin. She wants to walk about a bit more if she can as this will help combat the swelling in her legs. However, knowing Mum as I do, I know that she will try to do too much too quickly. She needs to take it slowly and I know that she will find this hard. Instead of taking baby steps, she will try and perform giant leaps for mankind. And although she is feeling better today, we must remember that a few days ago she nearly died. That is what chemotherapy does – it takes you to the brink of death in the hope that you will come back with bone marrow which behaves itself again. The idea – in layman's terms – is to reset your bone marrow. So although we smile and celebrate the daily improvements, it is difficult to overcome the other glaringly obvious signs of this disease: she is still hooked up to oxygen; she is still struggling to sit up on her own (or indeed move on her own); she doesn't stand up straight, instead standing with the stoop familiar to all hospital wards – the stoop of the very very sick; she tires easily and still falls asleep mid-sentence; her eyes are black from the weight of her glasses sitting on her nose; she needs help to walk and is taken for various procedures in a wheelchair. And I don't want to be the voice of doom so I (and Dad) smile and pretend that everything is fine (and hide the mirrors so that she can't see the state of her hair!).

And so to surmise…she seemed much more upbeat this morning but, as ever, things can change very quickly. So your continued thoughts and prayers mean a lot to us.

xxx

# Just Call Me Delia Smith
## 10 July

Today saw more improvement…hurrah!!! She not only went for a walk to the mini coffee shop near the ward, she also managed a picnic in the garden. The hospital food is appalling so she has asked for us to take food in. Today I took her piri piri chicken kebabs (with courgettes and cherry tomatoes), homemade tzatziki and crusty bread roll with gooseberry fool to follow. I'm pleased to say her appetite returned with gusto!!!

She went for another CT scan today as despite being on antibiotics since last Monday night, her temperature is no lower and this is puzzling them. However, she is not unwell with it so they are deploying 'watchful monitoring'…what you and I would term 'we'll wait and see what happens'. Her white cells are down again and her platelets are up from where they were when she was first admitted.

Signs are positive that she is fighting this and possibly doing well.

Also today she was fitted for her headscarves. Her hair is expected to fall out by next week (and is already thinning slightly – but not so that many people would notice) so she is now equipped with two scarves, one pre formed headscarf and one night time one. It was hard to see her in them but she looked so beautiful in them – she's chosen really bright ones and one that is made up of stunning autumnal colours – that I'm sure when her hair is finally gone, she will feel confident thanks to today's purchases.

Next Wednesday the wig lady will fit her – she has decided to go for the head of hair she has never had and get…I'll let that be a surprise! :)

xxx

# Looking Swell
## 12 July 2013

The last two days have seen a steady improvement – and a steady swelling of her legs. However, the more she moves, the less swollen she will be so she has been on a couple of walks (to the shop and into the garden for a bit.) The absolutely fantastic news is that she is allowed home on day release!!! Tomorrow afternoon she will be going home for a few hours. Being in her own house surrounded by her own things will make such a huge difference to her; and to Dad I think. She doesn't plan on doing anything once at home, other than sitting and resting, but she is so excited to be able to leave the hospital.

However, with the good news comes some not so good. Some patients with Acute Myeloid Leukaemia go into remission after chemo and only need chemo to beat the disease. Unfortunately, it would seem that Mum is not one of them. It is likely that she will have another two rounds of chemo and probably need a bone marrow transfusion. Obviously this is an upsetting prospect and is another blow, especially as she has been doing so well in the last few days. However, we will remain positive and hope and pray that if a transfusion is needed then a match will be found and found quickly. We will not worry about it just now; at the moment we just need to focus on her getting better and coping with this round of chemo. She is responding really well and her blood is doing what it should after chemo – her white cells are right down and the doctor is happy with the way things are happening. She will be very susceptible to infection as she has no immunity but that is not something to worry about today. (Maybe tomorrow.)

Your continued prayers and best wishes are, as ever, greatly received.

xxx

# Message from Mum

I feel well enough to do an update myself – I am feeling a lot better physically and have more energy. I finish the first round of chemo on Sunday and the hospital says I can go home for a couple of hours tomorrow and perhaps next week. Thank you for the overwhelming number of cards and messages, and for all your prayers and good wishes. The consultant told us that the nature of the leukaemia means that chemo alone is very unlikely to be enough. I will probably need a bone marrow transplant further down the line. So please keep praying for me – the staff in here are absolutely marvellous and I know I am in great hands. Please thank God for their skills. I do miss you all, but I am very vulnerable to infection for a while, so hope you will be patient a little longer before Ian and Ant arrange visits for those who would like to. I am not allowed flowers in hospital, but your cards and messages really cheer and support me when I am low, as does my bible!

Dee
(sent via email on 12th July 2013)

# Peaks and Troughs
## 13 July

Hi all,

So yesterday seemed so hopeful and she was so much better that today's news was, I'll admit, a bit of a blow. Although she was well enough to send out an enthusiastic and fairly positive email last night, shortly after she pressed send, her temperature spiked (the peak I refer to in my subject) and unfortunately it didn't come back down. She has a minor infection of some sort and this meant that today she was hooked back up to IV antibiotics and given a 2l blood transfusion. The result was that she was unable to come home. Although a minor setback in the grand scheme of things, it was still upsetting, especially knowing how much she wants to get home and spend time in her own house, surrounded by her own things.

However, she can't fight the infection because there is nothing in her bone marrow to fight it. This means that the chemo is doing its job so there is some semblance of a silver lining to this. (Even as I typed that, it felt like clutching at straws!!) There is still talk of her coming home at some point so it is only a very minor setback and at least she didn't come home and THEN get the infection – that would've had her worried about going back home in case it happened again.

Anyway she will not be brought down (the trough) by such a small infection – she will continue to fight and we will continue to support her in any way we can.

Love and prayers.

xxx

# A (Temporary) Change of Tone
## 15 July

Hi,

She got a day's release yesterday and today so spent three hours at home with my dad. She has already remodelled the flooring for the whole of downstairs and is planning radical changes to the garden. This may be news to my dad. She is also teaching Dad to cook; she sits on a stool in the kitchen and tells him what to do. No change there then. Anyway, back to the boring stuff…her temperature is okay again, although she had to return to the hospital by eight o'clock for her next dose of antibiotics (or in case her coach turned back into a pumpkin). Her bruises are dying down a bit apart from the ones under her eyes which are apparently caused by the weight of her glasses. She is less swollen than last week and her smile has made a welcome return.

We continue to have our ups and downs as the realities continue to hit home. Holidays that have been talked about and eagerly planned and anticipated are now being cancelled; visiting friends who should be causing flurries of cleaning and preparation are instead being emailed visiting times; milestones are (and will be) missed; and it hurts like hell. And although we know the support is there, I guess it's fair to say we are angry. We are angry at a lot of things and at the same time at nothing in particular. It simmers away in us, beneath the surface, threatening (but never quite managing) to overwhelm us.

Because ultimately this isn't fair. I don't care how strong she is…this just isn't fair. And that hurts. Yes she is strong and yes she is a fighter but some days we just ask ourselves 'where does being a fighter get you?'. And the answer is not yet apparent. But overriding the anger is hope. Hope that things will be made right. Hope that we will get through the anger (and I'm assured that it is part of the 'process' and is totally normal; for this reason I know we will all get through it, eventually.) and come through it unscathed.

BUT the anger doesn't spill over. Why? Because we have love, and we have the strength that you all give us, and we have faith. Faith that ultimately all will be right. She IS a fighter and that WILL get her through.

xxx

# A Wig and a Prayer

The past two days have seen Mum in her own house, albeit on the sofa, resting. Yes people, it's true, she's allowed out every day!!! At the moment she is allowed to come and go but she has to be monitored closely and the slightest hint of infection will see her confined to her room again.

Today the wig lady came. Despite my best efforts to persuade Mum that a long blonde curly wig was the way forward, she was not to be convinced. Luckily for her, I had anticipated this so had found a few styles I thought might suit and took her the pictures. She tried on three wigs, two of which were totally wrong. The third, however, was a revelation. She looked amazing. It's the hair she was always meant to have and it makes her look fifteen years younger. In fact if you weren't expecting to see her, you would probably walk right past her in the street!!! Dad's face was priceless when he saw her; it wasn't the style he expected her to go for so he got a bit (understatement) of a shock when she walked into the living room with it on. However, even he admits that it could have been made for her and that she looks fantastic in it.

As with all things there is a downside…to wear a wig well you have to have no hair. So next Wednesday at 9am the wig lady is coming back. And this time instead of neat boxes filled with confidence saving hair pieces, she will be bringing with her a pair of hair clippers. Her head will be shaved and the wig trimmed (or 'feathered' if you will) at the front to frame her face perfectly. As hard as it will be to see her without hair, it will be infinitely harder for her. As an alopecia sufferer, I can tell anyone that there is a terrible sadness in being able to see, and feel, your own scalp. It's one of the things that can completely crush your confidence and is something you have no control over. Hard as it may be for us to see her bald, it will be harder still for her to look in the mirror every day and witness the terrible reminder of the battle she is constantly fighting – good job this wig suits her so well as the boost it will give her confidence is immeasurable.

And so we move to the Leukaemia itself. All her blood counts are down which is good news as it means the chemo is doing as it should. Her bone marrow has been stripped and now we deploy 'watchful waiting' (The 'wait-and-see' I've mentioned before). In an ideal world, the bone marrow will start producing white cells by itself. In a few weeks she will have another bone marrow aspiration in order to check what is happening. If all is well, she can come home for a week or so after this. Then she goes back into hospital to start this process all over again. She will have (approximately) two more cycles of treatment and then we see about a bone marrow transplant. Although we now have an overview of the treatment we continue to take things one day at a time – it's all we can do. Too far ahead and it's too much to take in. Small steps is all we can manage; it's a strategy that's working so far.

Keep praying for us. For all these messages seem positive she still has a long hard fight ahead.

xxx

# BBQs and Besties
## 19 July

Hi all,

Today we had a BBQ. Mum came. As did one of her best friends and their family. It was amazing. Such a perfectly normal thing to do but oh so very special because she was allowed to be there. I never thought I would be filled with childlike enthusiasm because Mum was coming to sit in my garden and criticise my cooking/cleaning skills/bathroom cleanliness. But I was enthused; I couldn't wait.

And it didn't disappoint.

We cooked far too much food and we ate far too much food. We talked and argued and laughed and (at times and, hopefully, discreetly) cried. It was fabulous because she was there and it all had a feel of normality to it.

But the 'normality' didn't quite sit right: we knew better. Mum arrived in trousers and a long sleeved shirt. She is no longer allowed to sit in the sun as the chemo means she is more sensitive to UV rays. She wore a hat which suited her so much it was heart breaking – because Mum has never found a hat that suits her and now that this happens she finds the perfect shape and style. Go figure! And the worst bit? The announcement – made very quietly and only to me – that her hair has started to fall out. When she shakes her head, she gets 'a fall' of hair. And the bewilderment that goes with it. What should she do? Should she just bite the bullet and shave it off now? Should she wait until Wednesday for the wig lady to do it? Should she start wearing a scarf now or wait until it's gone? Answers on a postcard please. She thinks tomorrow will be the morning when she wakes up with hair on her pillow and this thought scares her. (Who wouldn't be scared?!) So we need to prepare and steady ourselves, ready to support her. For all we can say that there are worse things than losing your hair can anyone honestly say that they wouldn't mind? Because I couldn't. But Mum? She just worries about her hair falling in my food at the BBQ. She is an inspiration; albeit an exasperating one.

xxx

# Reception Called, They Want to Upgrade You

Hi all,

Yesterday Mum was allowed out again (this shouldn't change unless she gets an infection, in which case they will lock her back in and fill her with antibiotics) and she spent the day at home with Dad. I popped in with Lily and Alba which cheered her up (I think). When I arrived I found the house like the Marie Celeste – telly on, door wide open, slippers abandoned on the rug – and I nearly had a heart attack fearing the worst had happened and Dad had had to rush her back to the hospital. I decided to check outside before tearing off to NTH and lucky I did, because in the garden I found Mum, stretching over things to pick raspberries off the vine. After a few steadying breaths, I asked what she thought she was doing and was met with the response: "Your dad's at the shops as there's no food. Don't you start." She then proceeded to nearly trip over on her way out of the flower bed and cause my heart to jump right back into my mouth!!! (It turns out the abandoned slippers were Dad's protest at having to go to Tesco – his least favourite place after The Metro Centre.)

Anyway, after the near heart attack we had a cuppa and a nice chat and then I went on my merry way. Mum went back to hospital and all was (and is) fine.

Today she was moved rooms. This is because all the rooms share a bathroom with the room next door (Jack-and-Jill style.) The policy is two men or two women share a bathroom but due to circumstances for the past few days the room next to Mum has been occupied by a man (Gasp in horror – who'd have thought it?!). They have now moved

Mum so that the poor bloke next door can use his bathroom again and Mum is sharing with another woman. I'm sure there's an excellent medical reason (cross contamination etc.) for this but, to be honest, it seems a bit…well, daft. Anyway, she's now across the corridor from her other room. Hopefully it is cooler than the last one. And hopefully I don't go to her old room on autopilot tomorrow. That could become awkward!

xxx

# You Don't Know
# You're Beautiful
## 22 July

Fabulous news today! Mum is not only allowed home but is also allowed, wait for it, TO SLEEP IN HER OWN HOUSE!!!!! WOO HOO!!! :) Apologies for the slightly over exuberant start to this message but it is fantastic news for her. Not only is the hospital bed fairly uncomfortable (as Mum grumbled the other day, "I've slept in a Tempur mattress for a long time, Ant. This bed just does not measure up!") but as anyone returning from holiday can tell you – there's nothing like sleeping in your own bed to ensure you get a good night's sleep. Hopefully she will get a full night's sleep and be rested in the morning.

When I spoke to her earlier (I won't go to see her tonight as I returned to work today and so have come into contact with so many germs I hate to think what I might catch, let alone someone with no immunity at all!!!), she sounded tired and admitted she was having a bit of a down day. Her hair is falling out in handfuls and this is obviously distressing for her. Although Mum would be the first to admit that her hair would not be described as one of her best attributes, it is still HER hair – and so losing it is very difficult. She feels very self-conscious and although she tried on one of her scarves it was, in some ways, more distressing than the bald patches. Who can say why? Maybe it's the knowledge that this is how she will look for the foreseeable future (still beautiful to me. I'll love her no matter how much hair she does, or doesn't, have as will Dad obviously!), or maybe it is just that, other than the bruising which is now beginning to fade, this is the big outward signal to the world that she is ill. Whatever it is, may she find it in her to stay strong and remember that inside, AND out, she is my BEAUTIFUL mum and she is loved by us all.

xxx

# Bald and Beautiful

Mum's head was shaved today. I was with her the whole time and it was one of the most emotional things we have encountered so far. She was so brave but I could tell that she was close to tears and scared. Her hair was very thin and I'll admit that it did look pretty pathetic before Sam (the wig lady from Hairtopia in Darlington) worked her magic. However, Mum transformed before my very eyes. I watched as Sam shaved off what was left of Mum's hair and then I watched as Mum became truly beautiful. When Sam had finished, Mum looked (and I am not kidding here – I promise you it was as much of a shock to me as it will be to you) like a cross between Sinaed O'Connor (minus the chest and arm tattoos) and Annie Lennox. Sam had used a guard on the clippers so Mum has about 1/2 a cm of hair left. Although this will fall out over the next few days, the lack of length will mean less stress on the follicles and so less pain for Mum (her scalp has been very tender for the past week.) It also makes the whole thing more humane somehow. Then she put her wig on and it was trimmed to frame her face perfectly.

Although we all know that at some point she will be totally bald, she will be more used to the lack of hair by then. And she looks just as beautiful without her wig as she does with it. In her own words, "I might feel okay answering the door without my wig. Maybe. One day." I wanted to hug her so hard and tell her just how amazing I think she is. But I didn't. Because if I had, she would have cried which would have set me off; and we've all cried enough as it is. But I can tell you all – my mum is amazing. She is beautiful, courageous, brave, strong and fragile. She is fighting this with more dignity than I could ever imagine and she does it with a humbleness that, at times, renders me speechless. She doesn't want anyone to tell her how brilliantly she's doing – she just wants to be well again. But I want to tell her – and all of you, and everyone else in the world – that she is bloody brilliant and I love her very much.

Enough soppiness. After the head shaving, it was time for another IV drip of anti-fungal medication, then the ward rounds. Her consultant had a fair bit of information for us, so here goes:

It will be at least 2 weeks until she has another round of chemotherapy. There is still no sign of her bone marrow producing white blood cells but they are (hopefully) expected any day now; certainly within the next 10 days. Once the white cells appear they will do another bone marrow aspiration to see what levels there are. While the consultant was there, I asked why Mum had to have more chemo. If – I reasoned – her bone marrow showed 'normal' levels, why do they need to strip it again and again? The answer was because when looking at blood tests and bone marrow, 1 out of 100 Leukaemia cells might be seen with the naked eye. So even if the sample LOOKS like all the Leukaemia cells are gone, they probably won't be. So to remove the risk of the Leukaemia returning they do more rounds of chemotherapy in order to ensure that the Leukaemia cells are eradicated.

Whilst at home, Mum must (wherever possible and within reason) stay away from infection. Her temperature was up to 37.7 today. If it goes any higher, she needs to ring the hospital and go straight back in.

Her red cells and platelet levels are good. Yesterday she had a platelet transfusion which means that she didn't need to have one today.

She is not yet an outpatient (although the nurses seem to disagree and they are a scary bunch.) Although there are others who may need the bed, her consultant is not ready to give it away yet. He thinks it is important that her room is there just in case she needs to come back in – because she will have to come back in very, very quickly. That's a sobering thought and a timely reminder that although she is doing fabulously at the moment it can all change in the blink of an eye. We just have to hope and pray that it doesn't.

xxx

# Is It Just Me or Is Everything...?

I'm not an optimist – I never have been. My mantra has always been: 'A pessimist is never disappointed, merely pleasantly surprised.' However, sometimes something happens that makes me think, *Well that's just s\*\*t.* That happened today. I just called Mum to enquire as to the whereabouts of a picnic basket and two fold-y chairs, only to be told that she was back in hospital and they have no intentions of letting her out today. The reason? She had A REALLY BAD NIGHT. Awful in fact. She got no sleep whatsoever and was in so much pain that she could barely walk in to the hospital at 8am this morning. (I think they may be cross with her. I bloody hope so. I'm furious!) The reason for her bad night was her back. The sight of the bone marrow aspiration is still causing her pain and discomfort but last night, try as she might, she could not get comfortable. The painkillers they had given her were making no difference (the first thing they did this morning was change them to Tramadol!) and her temperature has gone up to 38 degrees.

So they have sent her for an x-ray to try and determine the cause of pain. Mum has a history of back problems and she suspects that her back has 'gone' again and that's why it is all so painful. We will see. She is currently waiting for the ward rounds to see what they say. She is sending Dad home after the consultant has been then he's going back this afternoon. My aunty is going in as well (she had cancer some years ago so is helping immensely when Mum needs to ask someone, who isn't the consultant or me and Dad who are both clueless, questions.) So I am not. I asked if she wanted me but she is exhausted and the Tramadol makes her sleep so she said she would rather see me tomorrow. Instead I am going to ferret out the flaming picnic basket and chairs and go to the park to watch *Babe the Sheep Pig* with my gorgeous family. And, barring being at Mum's bedside, there is nowhere I would rather be tonight. I just hope it doesn't rain* – that WOULD be s**t!

Xxx

*It rained. Obviously!

# Pretending Is Hard

Mum seemed very down today. I guess the 'one step forward, two steps back' nature of this battle is starting to get to her a bit. She has definitely contracted an infection and is now receiving specific antibiotics to target it. She is also being given anti-fungal medication, saline fluids and is scheduled for a blood transfusion.

However, the transfusion cannot happen until her temperature comes down. This is happening, but slowly.

The mood in her room today was... flat. She's back to falling asleep mid-sentence and back to being exhausted. Her sense of humour seems to have (understandably) disappeared. Her new room is hotter than the last one and because it's on the other side of the corridor she cannot open the window due to building works and risk of further infection. She has lost weight – a lot – in the few weeks she has been ill, but instead of being cause for celebration it merely highlights that all is not well. If anything it gives her a haunted, hunted look; as though this disease is literally hunting her down and stalking her every step. All semblance of vanity is gone in front of Dad and I now. A mixed blessing, I feel. On the one hand it means that she is too tired and too uncomfortable to bother (I feel like that with a cold so it's certainly no surprise). On the other hand, it means that she is comfortable enough with Dad and I that she doesn't need to pretend.

We've all become good at pretending. On a morning when I wake up, I pretend that I'm going to have a 'normal' day and that today she might get the news that actually it was a misdiagnosis and she's perfectly fine. Then later, when I get to the hospital, I pretend that I am not scared. I do this because it seems like a very small thing to do for her when she is going through so much. Then when I leave, I pretend it doesn't hurt and that I don't want to climb on the bed and cuddle her and never leave her. Then when I get home I (try) and pretend to my family that I am fine and that she is doing brilliantly and there is nothing to worry about. Tony pretends not to see me cry (and I love him for it). Dad and I pretend that there is not a big white elephant in the room whenever we talk about her treatment and her future; we pretend that there is no possibility that she could die. But that's the reality. And on days like today, when it is almost too much effort for her to smile, it's hard to avoid. It sits in my heart like a stone, cloaked by fear. She can't die, she has to get better because I'm not ready to face the world without her. Putting it simply, I don't know how. And I don't want to know how. Not now. Not ever.

xxx

# A Possible Turn-Up for the Books

So, better news today. Mum was SO much better than yesterday, in spirit as well as health. Her platelets have stabilised so she does not need platelets or a blood transfusion today. And the HUGE news is that for the first time her neutrophils are 0.1. This means that there is a possibility that her bone marrow is starting to produce white blood cells. We are trying not to get our hopes up yet as it needs to be confirmed by a second reading tomorrow and could just be a false alarm. But it is difficult not to feel pleased. We grasp, and cling to, any positive signs. She still has a temperature and so they give her paracetamol to try and bring it down. However, this makes her sweat (sorry Mum) so it can be very uncomfortable, especially at night when she is trying to sleep – especially since she can't open a window in her new room due to the aforementioned building works. However, as the Sister said today, "We've not got your temp down to 'normal' yet. Maybe 'normal' for you is just abnormal for everyone else."

We spent a lovely afternoon in companionable quiet – reading magazines, completing crosswords, snoozing (Mum in bed and me curled up on the chair). It was lovely. Normally, I despise that word; like 'nice' it tends to stick in my throat as somewhat lacklustre. But it sums up this afternoon perfectly. It was what it was; an afternoon spent in beloved company, doing not very much, just because we could. And it felt like time well spent. Doing 'nothing' with my mum is a rarity; normally one or the other of us is rushing round like a lunatic and often the time to just 'be' is quite simply not available to us. So today was a cherished afternoon. Just as, as a child, afternoons spent lying on a school playing field spotting shapes in the clouds was an afternoon well spent, so was today. If nothing else, this illness has taught me the following; it doesn't matter what you spend your time on as long as it is shared with someone you love.

xxx

# Life Is a Rollercoaster, Just Gotta Ride It

So I haven't written anything for the past three days and today I asked myself why. It took me a while to find an answer. It's because I couldn't decide what to write. On Monday morning, I felt quite upbeat and the post would have reflected that. However after a visit to see Mum I felt quite down (Monday was not a great day) so had I written the post on Monday night it would have been all doom and gloom. Tuesday morning was still doom and gloom but by Tuesday night (after an afternoon visit to Mum) I was considerably cheered. And I've realised that this is just one of the devastating things about Acute Myeloid Leukaemia; it is an emotional rollercoaster for everyone involved. It is appalling for Mum who has had to go through MORE procedures (such as the removal of her Hickman line) and it is appalling for Dad who has to watch her go through it while feeling totally powerless. Bringing in clean nighties and tasty nibbles is all well and good but realistically that's about as far as our practical help can go. We organise things – a cleaner for the house, people to do the ironing, visiting schedules, goodbye meals with departing friends – but what we actually want to do we can't. Because if we could we would climb under her skin and seek out every rotten leukaemia cell and kill them, quickly, efficiently, painlessly and PERMENANTLY. However, we can't so rather than dwell on this, we shall have to dwell on the positives, of which, for once, there are many! :)

Here we go…

The Hickman line was removed yesterday. It took an hour and a half to remove it and was painful at times. It was removed because they believe that it is the source of the infection she couldn't shake. It was badly swollen and painful but once removed she began to stabilise. Her temperature was stable through the night and she did not suffer the usual night sweats that seem to plague her recently. It also came down by a degree so they are all pleased with her.

Today's blood test results show that Mum's neutrophil count is up to 0.3 which means her body is producing white cells by itself – fan-bloody-tastic! :) Her platelets have also made a huge jump from 26 yesterday to 78 today. Again this is brilliant because her body is doing this on its own without the need for blood transfusions. And so for the best news…following this evening's antibiotics Mum can go home and stay the night. She needs to go back to hospital in the morning to have her bloods taken but, all being well, she will be switched from IV antibiotics to a course of oral antibiotics AND THEN SHE WILL BE DISCHARGED!!! Yep, that's right, she will be discharged and sent home for a week. After the week, she will need to have another bone marrow aspiration to see what is happening and then the next stage of her treatment will be decided. She will have to be readmitted for the next set of chemo but at least she will spend a chunk of time in her home surrounded by her things. AND who knows, maybe she can actually have some visitors at some point (if they can get past Dad.)

So, today I am feeling good. My mood is up and I can't wait to see her at home, where she belongs.

xxx

# She's Home

Fabulous news!!!

Yesterday went like clockwork so today Mum came home for good. On Tuesday she needs to go for an appointment at the day unit for bloods and assessment. Following this she will need a new Hickman line and then will start round two of chemo.

She is now taking oral antibiotics and has been discharged with a week's worth.

Wednesday's MRI scan shows two bulging discs, one of which is pressing on the sciatic nerve. The good news about this is that the back pain is not to do with the Leukaemia, just the historic back problems. Happy days! :)

She seems so much better than she did three days ago. I went round for a few hours this afternoon and she was a semblance of her old self – bossing Dad around, playing farms with Lily, laughing at Alba – which was a joy to witness.

But (and isn't there always a 'but' in these posts recently?) because I am not an optimist, I have taken it all with a pinch of salt. She IS better, and she IS fighting and today it would look like she IS going to win; her white cells are 0.3, her platelet count is increasing as we speak, her temperature is stabilising. But what will happen tomorrow? I don't know. No one does. We have to take it day by day because this illness can change in seconds. But for now she is doing well. And I know I sound like doom and gloom, and I wish that I didn't feel this way. But the post I wrote before this one, which was hearts and flowers and leprechauns and all things nice, didn't feel right. Every day is tinged with caution. Every day I value the time I spend with her. And the better she gets, the more I seem to err on the side of caution in these posts. Because when she is very poorly I only let myself think positively. As the old Persil advert stated – PMA (Positive Mental Attitude) will see you win anything. So we have a PMA every time we receive bad news. But is it just me that thinks PMA is bloody exhausting?! So on the days that she IS better I allow myself to think about the not so positive side…the 'what ifs' if you will. For example 'What if her temperature goes up again?'; 'What if she starts struggling with her breathing again?'; 'What if her neutrophils don't go above 0.3?'; 'What if her platelets start to fall?'. And the answer I keep coming back to? She'll go back to hospital and they will alter her treatment to target the 'new' problem. And then I don't let myself think beyond there. Because so far I (and Mum and Dad) have placed their trust in the specialists, doctors and nurses at NTH…and so far they have seen her right. They have been completely without fault and at times have gone above and beyond their jobs to soothe not just her worries, but mine and Dad's.

Without their tireless support and patience, I don't know where any of us would be. They have been truly amazing and a tower of strength for us all.

And so this is dedicated to the wonderful staff at North Tees Hospital, Stockton-On-Tees. They are amazing and without them we would not be the (semi) functioning family you see. Thank you. From the bottom of my heart, thank you.

xxx

# No Ifs, Buts or Maybes

Went to see Mum today. She was grand. She played farms with Lily, cuddled Alba and told me I needed to wash my hair. Pretty much back to normal. For this reason today's post is mercifully short. I have nothing to report. She's great. No ifs, buts or maybes. She's at home and she is happy. Here endeth the post! :)

xxx

PS: She's planning on going to church tomorrow.

# Without Friends We Are Nothing

Happy days are here again. Mum is out of the hospital and still doing well. We have a week and a half before the invasive treatment starts again (she is still on antibiotics but then so are about 65% of the population at any given time so this is nothing to worry about!) and we will enjoy it.

Mum made it to church this morning. I don't think there was a dry eye in the place. She walked in on my dad's arm and he looked so proud of her. It was very moving. Strangely (or perhaps not), she looked anything but sick. Her wig was styled to perfection and her raspberry jumper gave some colour to her cheeks. She looked amazing. And despite her pre-emptive warning that she would get emotional and cry, she didn't. Cry I mean. She was emotional – we all were – but the smile did not leave her lips for the entire service. Dad did not leave her side, and although his eyes shone with tears a few times (don't deny it Dad, it's more moving than I can ever tell you), the rest of him shone with pride throughout. As did I. I am immensely proud of them both. It is difficult to go to such a big gathering of people and not be overwhelmed; but they weren't. In fact the word I could use today is 'serene'. There was an aura of calm and peace surrounding them (as fanciful as that may sound.). I will pose two reasons for this, although I am sure there are more: One is that church is a place Mum feels at peace. Two is the love and strength she receives from her friends, many of who were in attendance this morning. The reason I can pose these reasons is simple…it's how I feel. Without friends we cannot beat this. Without friends we cannot continue to be strong. Without friends we are weak. Mum (I know) feels, and is, so very very lucky to be surrounded by friends; even if the treatment means that at time the surrounding has to metaphorical rather than literal, due to the lack of neutrophils!

So, to all friends out there; Mum's, Dad's, mine, old friends, new friends, friends we have not yet met – this one's for you. Thank you. We can't do it without you.

xxx

# News in Brief

Mum went back to hospital today for blood tests. The results show increases in neutrophils and platelets are steady so she is scheduled for another bone marrow aspiration on Monday. After the aspiration, she will be sent home to recuperate before a new regime of chemotherapy is decided and then begun. On the 'bright side' she gets to go home after the procedure before chemo, rather than staying in. Whoop de whoop. (Said with a sardonic twist of the mouth.) Isn't it funny how quickly our perception of 'good news' changes?

Other than the worry about the aspiration (those things are bloody painful and no one in their right mind would look forward to one.), she is doing well. She tires easily and her wig makes her very hot but she soldiers on. Her leg is still giving her trouble but that is not related to the leukaemia so I shall not dwell on it. All in all things are…fine.

xxx

# Pondering

Why on earth was that last post so hard to write?! I have puzzled till my puzzler was sore and all I could come up with was the following: Normally I am either super enthused or extremely emotional. Tonight I feel neither. Nor am I in anyway emotionally unstable. Everything just feels…fine. Which in itself feels wrong. It may only have been 4 weeks today since Mum was diagnosed but it has been an emotional rollercoaster. In the words of Ronan Keating 'we just gotta ride it' and we do so everyday. But the past few days have felt very strange to me. Because we know (as much as we can know anything) that for a week, at least, nothing is going to change. There is a lull and it has created a strange sense of unease in me. I'm no longer sure what to do with myself now that I don't have to rush around as much. Don't get me wrong. I'm still running around like a Tasmanian devil trying to fit everything in (show me a mother who doesn't, no matter what age her children are) but the urgency, the sense of 'if I don't get there, something dreadful might happen' has gone. I know that if I say I'll be at Mum's at three o'clock but I don't get there until four, it isn't the end of the world (although Dad will be cross.). And it feels so different. Almost like being in limbo. We're happy that she's at home but (I at least) feel like we're treading water. Moving neither forward in the immense battle, nor backwards. Just staying still, biding our time and waiting for the next skirmish to begin. If we won the first battle, the war is far from over. And I think I'm only just beginning to realise just how long this war might last.

xxx

# Here We Go Again

Hi all,

I've not written for a whole week because there was nothing to report. How lovely that has felt. Apart from a slipped disc trapping a nerve and causing her leg to fail to work properly Mum has been really good this week. (Even her and Dad's comedy fall outside the hospital today made them laugh rather than despair – oh how I wish I could get the CCTV footage from it. It would definitely earn £250 from *You've Been Framed!*)

In fact in terms of the Leukaemia she has been as good as we could have possibly hoped. The past week has been lovely: Mum has seen friends and been in her own house, she's gone out(!) for fresh air, she's even been allowed to have flowers because she is no longer neutropenic. It's been a happy time and we have enjoyed the 'normality' that at the beginning of the week felt so strange to us all.

Unfortunately, according to legend, all good things must come to an end and so today she went back to hospital for another bone marrow aspiration. This is so that they can check what is happening with the bone marrow and the different cells and use that information to decide on the next course of treatment. Which (in more practical terms) means that she will receive a phone call (or may have already received it) telling her when her next round of treatment will start. She will also be given a date for the insertion of a new Hickman line. The aspiration is a painful procedure and Mum having one today is a reminder that this battle has only just begun.

It's scary stuff but we've been there once and survived so we know we can do it again, but we may need that extra little bit of support in the very near future.

xxx

# Disappointment Came a Calling

Just got off the phone from Mum and the news is…disappointing; she goes back into the hospital tomorrow. They called her in today to discuss the results of yesterday's bone marrow aspiration and the alarm bells started ringing. They always tell you bad news face to face. The aspiration showed that the chemo had not worked as well as they were hoping and there are still an awful lot of Leukaemia cells. This means that tomorrow she will have a new Hickman line inserted and Thursday she will start the next round of chemotherapy. It will be different chemotherapy to last time as obviously the first lot didn't work very well. After that she needs a bone marrow transplant. It's all happening very quickly and although we feared the worst, we prayed for better news. What makes this news so hard to process is that we knew this treatment was going to happen but we didn't expect it quite so soon. It's scary because we knew that a bone marrow transplant was going to have to happen but we didn't think that it would be so soon. And now we see it cantering round the corner. Fast. I can't write anymore because my head is fuddled. I'm off to hug my mum.

xxx

# Rallying the Troops

Today was a horrible day. She is back in the hospital and it's really brought us low. We are back to the routine of visiting, bringing coffee, tasty nibbles for her to tempt her appetite, holding her hand.

Her new treatment path has been decided and is very full on. Mum had a new Hickman line inserted and is now in discomfort. She's been hugging an ice pack to the site all day, trying to numb it but to little avail. She has also had a port placed in the back of her arm through which she will receive daily injections which will hopefully kick start the production of white cells or platelets (she's not sure which). She will also receive a course of Tinzaparin injections which prevent blood clots (a possible side effect of one of the new chemotherapies she will be given.).

She will be given three different types of chemotherapy which will hopefully battle the Leukaemia cells more effectively. However they are much stronger than the last course of chemo; they have to be if they are going to work. And that means that Mum will be much more poorly than last time. I can't picture this. Having been there and seen her at her worst I cannot honestly imagine how she could get any worse. But they have promised that she will. She will be given other medications to combat some of the side effects of the chemo but how effective they will be differs according to each patient so there are no guarantees they will have any effect.

There is no dignity in illness. Tonight we could hear other patients suffering the effects of their treatment. It is awful because as much as I sympathise with the others, I am glad that, if only for tonight, it isn't Mum who was suffering that badly. And then I felt guilty, because everyone in there is someone's 'something': Mum; Dad; brother; sister; aunt; uncle; cousin; child. Everyone should have a family that cares about them, fears for them, cries for them, prays for them, watches over them and hopefully holds their hand. Mum is lucky that she has so many people doing all these things, and more, for her. But on nights like tonight, the hardest thing to do was to leave her room because, as I looked back to her lying on the bed, she looked small and lost and lonely and scared. And I KNOW she will be angry that I have written that because she is the strongest person I know and she was trying so hard to stay strong for me and Dad. But I wish she wouldn't. I wish she would let go. Because although I might not be able to do anything else, I can sure as damn it give good hugs. And though I gave her a hug, I still had to leave her: and tonight that was the last thing I wanted to do. Tomorrow feels like day one of the next stretch.

Today was mustering our strength and mentally preparing for what is winging its way towards us.

Bring on tomorrow.

xxx

# Sorry Isn't the Hardest Word

Today the chemotherapy started again. It's awful. She will be receiving chemo three times a day, every day. It drains her, renders her incapable of forming a sentence or even stay awake, makes her so poorly that we weep for her. We expect that family members will soon be contacted in reference to a bone marrow transplant because that is what we are careering towards.

Tonight Mum and I sat in near silence, both contemplating the next few weeks and the horrors that it will bring. There is so much that we want to say but at the same time there seems little point. She knows how much we love her and we know just how much that love is returned. When it boils down to it, what else is there to say? She dozed, fitfully, twisting to find a comfortable position. I read (or tried to read) a trashy book I found on the coffee table near to the nurses' station.

While sitting in near silence, I had a lot of time to reflect and I started to work out why this round is so much harder than the last. Last time round Mum was admitted and started her treatment within two days. We were given the diagnosis and then the nurses flung themselves into action. I realise now we were all in shock. Mum was suddenly so ill that at one point we didn't think further than the next hour; so the realities of the chemotherapy (and its side effects) didn't even begin to register properly. We were just so grateful that something was being done. But this time around, this time it's different. Even on the day she went into hospital this time round Mum seemed good. Barring the dodgy leg (which is still dodgy in case you were wondering) she seemed so much better. And it's a cruel blow that it was 'fake'. This time around we know how poorly she will get, but then we ALSO know that when she reaches that point she will CONTINUE to decline. We know that the next five days are going to be hour after hour of her getting more and more poorly, more and more tired, more and more physically and emotionally exhausted. And we are helpless because all we can do is watch. We will watch as she suffers side effects such as (but not limited to) nausea, vomiting, mouth ulcers, stomach upset, tiredness (ha!), hair loss…the list goes on. We can do nothing and then we have to leave her after we spend a day watching her and doing nothing to help. Because we can't because we are helpless.

So because we are helpless in respect to Mum, I have decided to do something that may help others. I have decided to host a 'Macmillan Coffee Morning' to raise money which will go to providing practical help for families affected by cancer. (After all, Leukaemia is cancer of the blood.) I am also looking into a recruitment drive for the Anthony Nolan Trust – the charity which matches donors to people who need bone marrow, blood stem cell or cord blood transplants. The more people sign up, the more lives can possibly be saved. But more about that later.

At 9.30pm, I had to leave. Mum was exhausted and I was at danger of falling asleep curled up on the chair. And then I discovered the hardest word to say. As a kid one of the hardest words to say is 'sorry'. Now it would appear that the hardest word is 'goodnight'. Tonight both Dad and I struggled to say it; we each tried for over an hour but didn't manage it. We started trying approximately an hour before we left and were still struggling as we walked out of the door. We didn't want to leave her, lying on the bed looking fragile and exhausted. We never want to leave her. So here it is:

Goodnight, Mum. Love you.

xxx

# Harder by the Hour

I just got back from the hospital after an emotional two days. Mum is in a steady decline thanks to the rigours of chemo and the agony of a bad back. Yesterday was a quiet day. Not much happened of any note – Mum slept, Dad and I did crosswords, nurses came and went. Today was a slightly different story.

When I arrived today, it was to be greeted with the news that Mum had had a fairly traumatic morning. She woke at around half six, was fine, brushed her teeth etc. and got back into bed. Soon after she began to experience 'strange' back pain.

When she could stand the pain no longer, she called one of the nursing staff and asked for some pain relief. Unbeknown to Mum, the pain she described raised alarm bells with the nurse – because it sounded very much like a heart attack. Over the next few hours she endured a battery of tests including ECG, ultrasound, blood tests and more. After an extremely tense morning the test results showed she had not had a heart attack. However, along with the flood of relief we felt, we also felt that familiar niggle of worry. Because if it wasn't a heart attack, then what was it? The answer is still unknown. There are numerous possibilities: Angina, Kidney stones, kidney infection, water infection, trapped nerve, slipped disc...the possibilities are endless (as the recycling adverts tell us.). And as yet there is still no definitive answer. When I left her, another doctor was doing yet more tests to see if they could determine the problem. This one seemed to favour the idea of 'stones', but who knows? It could be anything really. And one of the very scary things today was the realisation that it could very easily have been a heart attack; it is one side effect to the chemotherapy. So now we have something else to worry about; which is just what we need.

On top of all that was another development: Mum's legs aren't doing what she tells them. (Her words, not mine). Which to you and me means that she can't move one leg without using her hands or having someone else move it for her. This has been getting steadily worse for a while (see my other references to her 'dodgy leg'.) but we presumed it was a trapped nerve or something. Today though her other leg started playing up. Now this could be a side effect of whatever is causing today's back pain or it could be something else. Again, we don't know.

There's so much that we don't know. And so much that we don't want to know. Things we are scared to ask. Like 'Will this work?' and 'Why is she in so much pain?' and 'Isn't there anything else you can try?'. Because we are scared of the answers.

So we don't ask in the first place. We have enough to cope with at the moment without inviting more in. But at the moment I think the best word to use is 'overwhelmed'. We are overwhelmed by the speed of her decline. We are overwhelmed with the speed in which the staff respond to things that would appear to us to be fairly insignificant. We are overwhelmed by the work of the wonderful staff. We are overwhelmed by our own ignorance. We are overwhelmed by people's love and generosity. We are overwhelmed by the strength of our feelings: fear, anxiety, love, hope, disappointment, tiredness, ashamed (that we would dream of even acknowledging tiredness or fear with what Mum is going through). We are overwhelmed.

For the first time tonight I did what people have been urging me to do: I asked for help. Not for me, but for my dad. I asked my aunty to take my place in hospital when I left because I wanted someone to be there for Dad. Someone to hold HIS hand, to give HIM a cuddle, to tell HIM it would be okay, to make HIM cups of tea, to be there for HIM. Because at the moment he's there for me and Mum and I fear that he is being forgotten. And I know he won't be because I know how many people there are who love him and will support him. But I also know that Dad won't ask them to. I know because I won't. Heck, where do you think I get my stubbornness from?! We won't ask, rightly or wrongly, for a variety of mixed up reasons. Like we think we can cope. We don't want to be a pest. And the biggest one for me (and Dad I think) is that asking for help would mean admitting how bad things are. If we have to ask then it's bad. And if we don't ask then it can't be that bad. That probably sounds ridiculous to many of you and it probably is; but I understand what I mean. And tonight I had to ask and my aunty was amazing. No questions asked, there in a flash, hugs all round, hands held, smiles restored (for now.)

People will always offer but sometimes accepting help can be too painful.

Sometimes you need people to barge in, take the coffee pot out of your hand and make the damn thing for you (like someone did for me this morning). Because that way you're not admitting how bad things are, so bad that you need support. You're just admitting that you have really bossy friends.

xxx

# Emotionally Wrung Out

Last night was terrible for Mum. She was the worst we have seen her and the nursing staff were very scared. She was in excruciating pain and ended up having a morphine patch. This works in a similar way to a nicotine patch: it releases a slow, steady, constant amount of morphine into the body and this helped to control the pain she was feeling. She had her stats checked every fifteen minutes – this should tell you how critical her condition was.

However, she stabilised and then improved so we relaxed a little.

Today started off okay. She was a little confused and couldn't think of words but this was attributed to the morphine. However, at around about seven o'clock, she began to decline rapidly. It turns out that her oxygen saturation levels were very low. Her pulse was through the roof and her breathing was very shallow and very rapid. She was given various levels of oxygen but eventually was given 100% oxygen through a face mask. By this point she was confused, very agitated and not herself at all. We were introduced to yet another doctor who, it turned out, works in ICU (Intensive Care Unit). We were informed that unless she improved or stabilised, Mum would be moved to ICU in order to better increase her saturation levels. Blood was taken from her wrist and tested and then she was given an hour to improve. After an hour, she was tested again and the doctors were satisfied with the results. Mum was allowed to stay on Haematology for the night. BUT…and it's serious…if there is any change for the worse in her condition, she will be going straight to

ICU – the preliminaries have been done, she is in the system, do not pass go, do not collect £200.

So Dad and I left at 9.30pm, exhausted but happy that she is in the best place possible, with the best staff looking after her. I can't begin to express what emotions we have been through; suffice to say she is, for tonight, stable and for now that is enough.

xxx

# Positive Signs

Short post tonight. Following the dramas of Saturday and Sunday I am pleased to announce that the last two days have been relatively mundane. Yesterday she spent much of the day drifting in and out of sleep. The morphine patch did its job and took the pain away so that when she was awake she was able to read the paper, attempt crosswords and scowl at Dad and I. As I remarked to the nurses, "She must be feeling better; she's back to being bossy."

Today she had rallied even more. She went for a CT scan and the results were fine; her temperature is coming down and she is more herself. Tonight we watched *The One Show*, *Eastenders* and *Holby City*. She was well enough to shout at a few of the characters and demand, "Well why are they doing that?!", "What did she think will happen?!" and "Oh why do we bother watching this rubbish?!" (amongst other things).

I'd say she's definitely better than the other day.

xxx

# Register Now

Chemo has finished!!! Now we just have to wait and see what happens. She still has to have blood transfusions (she had two today), antibiotics, various other medications and fluids and has a catheter (not pleasant) so that she can have total bed rest. She also has a white plastic boot which she has to wear when in bed; two hours on, two hours off. This is to help her 'drop foot'. Sounds great doesn't it?!?! But if it helps then she mustn't complain.

Today she was really grumpy and shouted at us. She then demanded food from Marks and Spencer. Both of these things are good signs that she is improving; and she is so much better than Sunday and Monday. But before we all jump for joy and think she is on the mend I must say this: it is all relative. She is better than she was but that's because she couldn't have got much worse. She nearly ended up in Intensive Care so anything is an improvement. But in terms of being 'better', well it will take a long time before we can ever use that word. She needs a bone marrow transplant. Until she has that, she will not be able to beat this. And there's no guarantee that a match will be found. We are waiting on the results of test to determine if one of her sisters could be a match and if they are then it will be fantastic. But if they aren't then we will need to look to the national register. And unlike the thousands upon thousands of people who give blood, there aren't that many people (relatively speaking) who are registered bone marrow donors. The process now is much easier and MUCH less invasive than it used to be yet it is less publicised than blood donors.

So to all you wonderful people who ask on a daily, if not hourly, basis, "What can I do to help?", the answer is simple:

Follow the link below and register to be a bone marrow donor. It is quick, it is easy and it might just help a family/person in a similar situation to us.

*http://www.anthonynolan.org/What-you-can-do/save-a-life/Online-application.aspx*

xxx

# Happy Birthday to You!

Happy birthday to you,
Happy birthday to you,
Happy birthday dear mu-um,
Happy birthday to you!!!
Hip, hip... Hooray!
Hip, hip... Hooray!
Hip, hip... Hooray!!!!!!

No prizes for guessing what day it is today! Took the girls in to see Mum and I think that was the best present we could have given her (although she seemed pretty happy with her scarf and other bits and bobs.). Her smile, when Lily walked in proffering her handmade card and gift, lit up the room. She's been worried that the girls would forget her, but how could they? She is so important to Lily and has been a constant in her life from day one. There is no way that she will (or can) be forgotten. Lily asks about her every day and made her a card, without prompting, 'just to cheer her up'. A slice of cake each and lots of smiles, hugs and chit chat and we were on our way again; short and sweet. Just as it needs to be when there are a few of you because she tires so easily.

It is difficult when there are children. As an adult, I struggle to comprehend half of what is happening so I know how confusing this must be for her grandchildren. Luckily Alba is too young to understand but for the other three it is difficult to get their heads around the fact that one day Grandma was there, cheering them on at sports day, and the next she was in hospital, very poorly and for fear of infection they couldn't be taken in. And so crops up another side effect of this disease...children often just don't get it. We have told

Lily that Grandma is sick, she has something wrong with her blood and the doctors are trying to fix it but it will take a long time. To me this seems sufficient. But it doesn't stop the barrage of questions that arrive on a daily basis. "What medicine are they giving her?", "Will she be better for my birthday?", "Does it hurt?", "Can I see her?", "Will I ever get to stay there again?", "Why can't I stay with Grandee?". And although the temptation is to snap and say, "Stop asking so many questions!" I *try* to answer her as honestly as I can without scaring the bejesus out of her. Because it IS scary for them and they DO need to be told. I just wish sometimes that I had the answers. Lily will not be fobbed off with "We'll see" or any variation. She wants to know and is flaming persistent! I see a bright future as a lawyer/solicitor ahead of her at this rate.

So I try to find a balance – between telling the truth and telling too much. It is a fine line, and one I manage possibly 2 times out of 10; but hopefully I will get better with practice.

Anyway, Dad is having dinner with her tonight; a birthday picnic if you will. Which will be lovely despite the surroundings.

Happy birthday Mum. May next year be totally different.

xxx

# What a Difference a Day Makes

I went away on Monday morning. We went, two adults and two children, to Northampton to stay with one of my best friends (and godmother to both my girls). She's just moved house.

I have never felt so guilty in my entire life. Making the decision to leave while Mum is still in hospital was, honestly, one of the hardest I've had to make in a long time. As much as my heart, mind and body were crying out for a recharge, I was undecided as to whether I could, with clean conscious, do something as selfish as take time out. Time just for me to do what I wanted for a change. The reason it was so hard a decision was quite simple: How could I admit that I needed time out when Mum is going through something so difficult? And suffering it with such dignity and so little complaining. In the end it was Mum who urged me to go: She clearly knows me better than I know myself. It was heaven and the best medicine I could have taken (even though I refused to acknowledge that I needed it.) I have returned feeling fresher and rested and ready to continue my support for her in any way I can. I just wish it was as simple for her and Dad.

Tonight our church held a prayer vigil for her. From 6-10pm the church was host to most of the usual congregation. People came and went, music was played, prayers were said and support was shown. Mum knew nothing about it until the other day and it really touched her (she cried tonight when I was telling her about it.) It was such a beautiful thing to see and a beautiful thing to do. The support shown for Mum tonight – the love shown for her – was immense. I would say "Here's hoping it helps" but I think it already has; it's helped all the people who attended, people who feel impotent to help, who want to help and can see no way of doing so. It's helped people who want her to know how much they care; who want us to know how much they care. People who find solace and peace in the church. And I cannot express to all those who went how much it means to me, Dad and, most importantly, Mum.

Back to Mum…she is doing very well, in so far as she can be. In fact I can't believe how much better she looks since Sunday!!! Her potassium levels are low and so she is being given three huge bags of fluid with potassium in. This is making her swell again. But at least swelling is preferable to some of the other side effects she has experienced before now. Her foot is still causing problems so she has to have a splint in her shoe for much of the day. She is also having physio to help her 'dodgy' leg (which in turn is causing the floppy foot situation – the leg, not the physio.) She is still having platelet infusions and other 'stuff' (which is too medical and technical to get into right now.) but her appetite is back (Brilliant sign) and today I saw the biggest sign yet that she is improving; she had her wig on!!! It has been MIA for the past three weeks and it was so lovely to see it return. It makes her look so much better because it brings colour to her face. Mind you, the smile smeared across her face may have helped as well!

Dad took her to the café for a coffee today – he pushed her in a wheel chair. I can only imagine the clip of the pair of them; but strangely I think it would have looked at worst endearing, at best heart-warming. I will explain this no further, other than to say the pair of them never fails to make me smile with their Laurel and Hardy-esque double act.

She has asked me to take the time in to tell people that she has no access to the Internet while in hospital. She can't get emails, Facebook or anything else. She is also not yet up to replying to messages sent to her. She appreciates them immensely and they bring her much joy when she hears them, but please don't be offended if she doesn't respond to them. She also sends everyone her love. To which I will add my thanks.

Thank you all for your continued love, prayers and support.

Much love

xxx

# Short and Sweet

Minor panic tonight. When I called Mum to tell her we wouldn't be in until the morning, she countered with: "Oh, well tell your dad my temperature spiked a little while ago and they seem quite concerned. I've been for a chest x-ray, had blood tests and am waiting on the results of both." Needless to say Dad and I hightailed it to the hospital. By the time we got there the x-ray was back and showed that there was nothing wrong with her chest and her temperature had begun to come down. So panic over. She is 'fine' (relatively speaking). There is nothing new wrong with her and she is still doing better each day. Because of the commotion she missed tea so ate a cream scone instead. That, I feel, speaks volumes.

xxx

# Make Time

Another scare last night. Mum became tachycardiac during the night (which means she had an abnormally high heart rate.) There was some concern and many doctors in and out. Luckily, it has been resolved – the doctors think that it has happened because she has had so much fluid over the last few days and it is making her heart work harder than normal. They gave her a diuretic to help remove some of the excess water from her body and once it had taken effect, her heart rate slowed. This morning they started her on antibiotics again, just to be sure. Hopefully, it won't happen again.

The broken night meant that she was tired today. We popped in for a quick visit, taking Lily and Alba with us. They seemed to cheer her up immensely. (Tomorrow will be a longer visit because I go back to work on Monday so it will be all change.) She looks so much better that it sometimes slips my mind just how ill she actually is. She looks amazing in comparison to a week ago and it struck me again today just how up and down this journey is, and just how hard that is on all of us.

I didn't go to see her yesterday because it was a bit manic in our house for one reason or another. It's really hard not to go in and see her; to admit that I don't have time. Because I feel I should always MAKE time. There is no excuse. I know that all of you reading this will be shouting at me, telling me not to be silly, that I must take time for myself and for my family, spend time with the girls and with Tony, recharge my batteries so I can better support Mum. And as much as I know that on the one hand you are right, my response would be that Mum IS my family and she is the one who needs me right now.

I know it sounds as though I am being self-indulgent and stubborn, and in a way I am. But even when you know people only want the best for you it is still hard sometimes to make them understand my need to be busy – rushed-off-my-feet busy. I fill my days with as many tasks as I can because then by the end of the day I know I will be physically exhausted, as well as mentally drained. It guarantees me sleep. On the few days I have not been dead on my feet by bed time, I have lain awake thinking. And as any insomniac will tell you, four in the morning is hideous at the best of times; when the worst case scenario is playing on a loop in your head it is bloody unbearable. Most days I don't want to think more than an hour ahead. Chunking my day up means that I get through it. Empty time weighs heavily on me because I no longer know what to do. The very idea of 'relaxing' is laughable; if I let my guard (and shoulders) down enough to even begin to relax, the emotions threaten to overwhelm me. The unsayable thoughts and fears creep in and before you know it I am drowning in a sea worry and fear; unable to articulate what I am feeling; unable to comprehend the huge fight still ahead. So I look like I haven't slept properly in a month (I haven't), my hair is lank regardless of what I do to it, my skin is terrible, my cheeks dry from the salt in my tears, my eyes sore from the same; and I just don't care. I yawn my way through the days, lurching from one visiting session to another; arranging everything around those two hours I will spend in the hospital room with Mum. Because, for now, those two hours a day are the most important thing.

It is such a shame that it takes such an awful thing to make you step back and take stock. We spend our days rushing everywhere, rushing through things, eating on the go, never coming to a complete halt, never really looking at what is happening and either appreciating it or realising the impact it will have. But during those two hours a day with Mum – where we often do nothing more than sit in silence, smiling at each other and holding hands – I find myself at peace (or the closest thing to it.) I am with my mum, showing her my love and support, demonstrating her importance to me, to all of us. The very fact that Tony arranges it so that I can be MIA for two hours demonstrates his love for us. So you see, I feel terrible when I say "I don't have time". Because in the grand scheme of things, what is more important? What can I honestly say is more important than spending time with my mum? Nothing.

So I will continue to look sleep deprived. I will continue to yawn at five-minute intervals. And I will continue to make time. Because sometimes actions speak louder than words.

xxx

# Baby Steps

Mum was meant to go to the Freeman yesterday to have an initial consultation about the bone marrow transplant. (We still don't know if there is a donor match for her so we continue to live in hope. We pray and pray for news, even though we know that Mum will be the last person to hear thanks to the procedures they have in place. She will not be told at this consultation if there is a match...I don't think they've even got that far yet.) Unfortunately, the meeting was cancelled, due in part to the fact that Mum is still on oxygen a lot of the time. She would have had to go via ambulance and it was eventually decided that it would be better for her to go on Thursday and aim to get her off oxygen by then so that Dad can drive her there in their car. She has done amazingly well with weaning herself off the oxygen and has spent a lot of time without it. Admittedly she doesn't do very much other than sit in her chair and bark orders at us but this in itself is an achievement. Dad and I are thrilled that she is getting angry at us; it means she is becoming some semblance of her former self. She goes for walks – very short walks. She still has a splint in her shoe (the dodgy leg remains) and needs a zimmer frame. She struggles to get in and out of a chair and cannot walk too far without tiring. Wherever they go she needs a wheelchair. So it's fair to say the news is...mixed.

Other than this there is very little to report. Last week she got very very ill. This week she is marginally better. Her meds are a little mixed up because the cannula in her hand was not inserted properly so some meds have not been getting into her system as effectively as they could. This is not a huge issue but it was very uncomfortable for her as they tried to insert a new line into her hand. She gets a little stronger each day and for this we are grateful.

The other side to her getting ever so slightly better is that Dad can relax a little. And when he relaxes a little, he can admit how tired he is. We can both admit how tired we are. Tonight I left him with the instructions to open a bottle of wine, drink some while watching *New Tricks* and then get straight to bed. He needs to rest or he will be no help to anyone. (Are you reading this Dad?!?! If so then stop, turn off and go to bed!!!) I worry about him as much as I do about Mum for the simple reason that Mum has an army of professionals watching over her, keeping her on the right track, looking after her. Dad has me. And I am not there enough for my liking. However, we muddle through and do our best.

As ever, your prayers are greatly appreciated.

xxx

P.S. Mum's thrilled by all the letters. She is so touched that people have taken time to let her know what is going on. It makes her feel slightly less isolated. Thank you. xxx

# Sobering News
## 21 October

Yesterday Mum travelled to the Freeman Hospital for her initial consultation regarding the bone marrow transplant. It did not go as well as we may have hoped. There are two courses of action that Mum can take. One is to do nothing. They will arrange palliative care, monitor her and make her 'comfortable'. Two is to have a bone marrow transplant. This is not as simple as it may sound. There are numerous issues surrounding a transplant. It turns out that none of her sisters are a match so they will have to find an anonymous donor. There are two possible donors who they are 'looking into'. There is no certainty that they will be a match for Mum.

However, if one of them is a match then there are a lot of possible problems. The treatment will take place at the Freeman. She will be allowed only two visitors (me and Daddo) and she will be there for around six weeks. To start the transplant process she will receive a week's worth of intensive chemo, very similar to the stuff she had last time. Bearing in mind she nearly died last time around this is a scary prospect. Last time also damaged her heart. The transplant has a 15% risk of death for a 'healthy' (relatively speaking) patient; for Mum and her damaged heart the risk increases to 30-40%. Add to this the other possible complications: her body might reject the transplanted bone marrow, or her body may see the new bone marrow as a threat and attack it, it might not work. And even if it does work there is no guarantee that the Leukaemia will not return. This is the nature of the disease we are fighting.

So there you have it. There may be a donor, there may not. She may survive the transplant, she may not. She has to decide what course of action to take. It's shit.

She has another appointment at the Freeman a week on Monday. We'll know more then.

xxx

# One More Step

Mum received a letter last week. It was in response to her first appointment at the Freeman Hospital. It detailed the possible treatment routes she can chose from and the dangers associated with them. It was horrible to read; mentions of 'mortality' and 'palliative care' among other heart chilling phrases. There is a certainty that without further treatment she will die. The leukaemia will return and they will provide palliative care. There is a chance that even with treatment she will still relapse. There is a high risk of her dying whilst receiving the treatment. The future seemed bleak. Yesterday we were all sombre. Mum said she had "come to terms with the worst possible outcome". We discussed the pros and cons of the letter and I will admit that I cried. A lot. The horror I felt was indescribable. Any decision could be unnecessary; if they don't find a donor who matches her then there will be no discussion.

Today Mum had her second appointment at the Freeman. The news was surprising. They have found a bone marrow match. It is not a perfect match but the specialist is willing to use it. It is 'close enough'. This is a huge positive. Mum asked a lot of questions including what the chances are of her relapsing if she has the transplant. There is still a risk but it is not as high as the certainty of a relapse if she doesn't have it. The chemotherapy is strong and she will suffer when she has it, but again he is not worried about her heart being damaged further (which was a concern mentioned in the letter.). If she goes ahead with it then she will be in Newcastle for six to eight weeks. Dad and I will need to be with her. There is a lot more to this but to be honest a lot of it is a blur. Mum has three weeks in which to come to a decision. There is a date in mind – even pencilled in – but it is by no means confirmed. Either side can cancel at any time. If her current condition worsens then there will be no question of her having the transplant. And there is still that 40% risk of her not surviving the transplant.

However, before she can even begin to think about the practicalities of the transplant, her bone marrow needs to start doing its thing. And at the moment it is not. We are reassured that this is totally normal and that it can take a long long time but it worries us all the same. She is also having temperature fluctuations and is back on antibiotics, antifungals, platelets and a handful of other medications. She is doubtful that she will get out of hospital this week. We will keep everything crossed that these subside.

So there you have it; a mixed bag, I feel. But overriding everything else is that tiny ray of hope. It's the first positive we have had in a long long time. And a lot can still happen and Mum may decide that she can't face it again; that it is too big an ask; that she is just not up to the challenge. Or she may not. She has been through so much and no one but her knows if she can bear to go through it again. Whatever she decides we will be right there with her, by her side. Every step of the way.

xxx

# Another Step Backwards

Mum was told that she would be able to be at home this week. Sadly she caught another infection and is now in the hospital with all leave suspended indefinitely. Monday's appointment at the Freeman is looking doubtful. A CT scan shows that her lungs have deteriorated. Antibiotics are not fighting the infection she has. They have given her every type of antibiotic there is and none of them have worked. This is partly due to the lack of neutrophils. Antibiotics can only do so much and without any help from her body they are fighting a losing battle. They are now trying various combinations of antibiotics to see if that will help.

Mum is only allowed two visitors – me and Dad. And then only if we are fit and well. Although it is understandable that people want to see her it is unfortunate that most people (myself included at times) find it difficult not to touch her. Not to hug her, kiss her, hold her hand. Touching her is a way of proving that she is still here; it makes it so hard to believe that there could ever be a time when she is not around. But it is so dangerous for her. And no matter how many times we tell people, the moment they see her they forget. So they touch her and now she has another infection. Obviously it is not as simple as that – there are a lot of things that could give her an infection. But one thing I know for certain is that if less people touched her then her chances of contracting an infection would be greatly reduced.

So if there are any messages you would like to give Mum then can you please pass them via me? I will be trying to get in to see her every day although she is tired and slightly snappy. She tires easily and I don't want to exhaust her. But, as ever, she likes to hear news from 'the world outside the hospital'. She can't respond to emails/Facebook messages/every text message as she doesn't have an internet connection (or the energy). Anyway, as I have already said, Monday's appointment is looking doubtful. I have no idea where that leaves Mum in terms of a transplant but something tells me it is not boding well. A negative post, I guess, but I can only report what is happening. Another step backwards; another punch in the stomach; another obstacle in her way. I hope and pray for more positive news soon.

xxx

# No-Vember Fundraising

So, in order to fundraise (yes again) for the Anthony Nolan trust, Tony and I are giving up alcohol for November. Please sponsor us. The more we raise, the more we can help this fabulous cause.

Please, please, please sponsor us!

xxx

# It Wasn't a Huge Surprise

So yesterday's appointment at the Freeman was cancelled. No huge surprise but a setback nonetheless. Mum wasn't up to the journey and is still struggling to fight this infection. She is on various antibiotics and they are not working as yet. She also still has pneumonia.

Last night was a bad night for her. She slept very little (if at all) and is still suffering with sweats that come with the infection. It is pretty awful for her. Add to this the fact that after they took out one of her cannulas today, they came back to find a pool of blood on the floor where she was bleeding out and you'll see how just how this week has started.

Let's just hope it does not continue like this.

On a more positive note, Mum has decided that if they will do the bone marrow transplant then she will have it. That all sounds a but/if/but/maybe but you'll see why soon. If she doesn't fight the infection there is a chance they won't do the transplant. If they don't do the transplant, there is a chance that she can't beat the infection. Catch 22.

So there it is. Very basic post with no emotions today. Emotions are too hard. Right now I am functioning. Best that can be said really.

xxx

# Ohhhh Matron

Mum had a good night last night. She slept soundly; so soundly she slept through breakfast. No bad thing given the travesty it has been the past few weeks. For some reason she never gets what she orders. It has become a running joke; a farce that seems out of place in a hospital and more in keeping with 'Carry on Doctor'. I half expect Barbara Windsor to wiggle her way through the door, tray held aloft and giggles abounding. One day she ordered scrambled eggs, tomatoes and mushrooms followed by fresh fruit salad. She got mushrooms and tomatoes, no eggs because none had been sent for any patient and two Weetabix with full fat milk. Another day she ordered Weetabix and semi-skimmed milk, toast and a yoghurt. She got an omelette and a banana. It is beyond ridiculous. She now keeps a tub of muesli on the side and has that for breakfast instead of what arrives.

When I left tonight she was waiting for the on call doctor to come and insert a new cannula. She has been having some trouble with the one that was in so it has now been removed. Thankfully there were no dramas this time. I got the full story of 'the other cannula' tonight: The nurse removed the cannula, applied pressure, stuck a wad of gauze over it to continue the pressure and all was well. Mum then fell asleep. At some point she must have bashed her hand because she was awoken by the feel of warm liquid dripping very quickly down her hand. When she opened her eyes, the bed covers were covered in blood, as were her sheets and pillows; her hands resembled Lady Macbeth's. Peering over the edge of the bed, she discovered a 2ft wide pool of blood on the floor. That's when she realised that she was still bleeding rapidly and the pool was spreading. A nurse came in and nearly went into cardiac arrest before three more rushed in and got to work. So no drama then.

Anyway, she was (possibly still is) waiting for a new one to be inserted when I left. They removed the other one while I was there, just in case she started to bleed again. Not sure what they think I would have done; let's hope I never have to find out.

So there you go, no progress to tell you about per say, but (I hope) a small insight into the day-to-day life of a hospital patient. Carry on nurse...!

xxx

P.S. MUST state that this is in no way a reflection of the superb work done by the ward staff. They are AMAZING and I can't even begin to contemplate where we would be without them.

# What I Think
# You Already Know

This may seem a slightly random post but sometimes that's just the nature of the beast. Today's post is a list; a list of things that I think people already know but they may not. The reason for this list is that in the past few weeks a number of questions have arisen and I have thought that people should already know the answer. However reading back through the blog it seems that some of the more basic things have slipped through the net without me having actually posted them. So here you go, in no particular order: My list-of-things-I-think-you-already-know-that-you-may-not-already-know.

1. Mum is not allowed flowers. The water that they stand in is the perfect breeding ground for bacteria and infection.
2. She is allowed silk/fake flowers. Please feel free to send her some to cheer up her room (via Dad or I, obviously).
3. She has pneumonia.
4. She can't walk.
5. At any given time, in the triangle that is Mum, Dad and myself, one of us is angry at one of the others. Except we're not really angry at each other; we're angry at Leukaemia. Which is very futile. So we turn it on each other.
6. She still has no neutrophils. (Or anything else for that matter. Her bone marrow is completely empty.)

7. To effectively fight infection she needs neutrophils. If they come back, then the bone marrow has produced them. If the bone marrow produces them, it will also produce platelets, which is good.
8. It MIGHT also produce Leukaemia cells. Which is bad.
9. She struggles to breathe.
10. She is allowed limited visitors – Dad and I. This is to limit the risk of infection.
11. She has no Internet access in hospital so in order to avoid a HUGE phone bill she only checks emails once or twice during the week, and only when Dad takes her phone home and 'updates' it over the home wireless.
12. She can't concentrate long enough to read.
13. She is allergic to one of the medications she is being given and is covered in an angry red/purple rash. It itches.
14. She has really dry skin.
15. She alternates between hot sweats and cold shivers.
16. Some nights she hallucinates due to the medication she is given.
17. She worries about us more than she worries about herself.
18. She still manages to raise a smile when recounting the farce that is breakfast.
19. She is still really bossy.
20. I cannot hug or kiss or touch her. I cannot hold her hand, stroke her face or rub her feet. I cannot take my children to see her and let them kiss her hello or goodbye. I cannot watch Lily show her what she made at school, because the very fact that she has been at school means she is an infection risk. I cannot watch with her while Alba rolls over or takes her first steps in front of her because Alba is an infection risk. I cannot watch my children crawl over her like a human climbing frame; like they used to. She is too frail and too fragile.

But the worst thing by far? I cannot lay my head in her lap and weep.

And that is all I want to do. Because that's what I've always done when things get tough. And she would stroke my hair and listen to my incoherent ramblings and make shushing noises and somehow an hour or so later everything would seem a little bit brighter. And even though I know everyone thinks I am doing really well keeping everything together, there is a gnawing ache in my chest that signifies something huge. It signifies that one day, very soon, I might have to be the one who strokes the hair and listens and shushes and makes things better. And I know that I won't do it half as well as she did. And I wish she could be doing it now.

xxx

# There Is a Glimmer

We have been knocked so many times that I almost daren't write this. Time and again hopes have been raised only to be dashed again. And what I am about to write is by no means definite or a sign of things to come or anything tangible on which to fix any hopes.

Today there is a glimmer of hope; tiny, unsubstantial, barely believable but a glimmer all the same. After weeks and weeks of no news or bad news this is something that I barely dare acknowledge. Mum's consultant at NTH has been liaising with the specialist at the Freeman and they have decided to try something to break the catch 22. They are going to give her 'Enhanced white blood cells'. This is a treatment that has been mentioned before but discounted due to the fact that patients often react hideously to it. However there has been a lot of research and work done to reduce the risks and recently there has been a lot of positive responses.

The reason white cells are so important is as follows: White blood cells are the part of the body that remove infection. Antibiotics and antifungals will (if you forgive the whimsy) bash the infection on the head and white blood cells then remove what's left. Neutropenic patients have no white cells and so although the medication bashes the infection down, without the white cells it will never be fully beaten. The decision to give Mum the enhanced white cells means that she is in with a chance of beating the infections which currently plague her. And if she can beat the infection then she can have the transplant. The treatment will start tomorrow.

So now you see the cause of my unease at the start of this post. I daren't believe that she may beat the infection because we have been close to the transplant before and then…well there is always an 'and then'. That's why I've stopped, or tried to stop, getting my hopes up. It really sucks when they get quashed – again. So I will end this post by taking a deep breath and repeating what I originally started with. There is a glimmer. And only time will tell where, if anywhere, it leads.

xxx

# And so It Begins

The treatment started yesterday. Mum's consultant was not rostered on yesterday but he came to work anyway and sat with her through the ten bags of enhanced cells (I can't remember the medical term for these but when I find out I shall let you know.). If she was going to have a negative reaction to them, then it would happen within five minutes of the infusion starting. I am pleased to say that Mum did not have any reaction yesterday. There were a lot of medical staff monitoring her, various staff from the ward, her consultant and the junior doctors among others.

This morning she was 'a lot brighter' according to Dad; 'a lot more chipper'. We are attributing this to the fact that SOMETHING is finally happening. For as long as I can remember, we have been waiting for something; white cells, red cells, temperature spikes to abate, test results, and so on and so on. This feels different. Under the guidance of various medical professionals Mum is having a different treatment – one that is not often given and so it feels different. Not every Leukaemia patient is given these cells and because she *is* it feels more proactive.

However (you knew it was coming!), this evening brought its own dramas. Mum had a HUGE temperature spike. When she has a temperature spike, she becomes very disorientated and can hallucinate; she loses her words and forgets what she has said. Tonight she also had violent shakes and memory loss: She forgot that she had had medication and when questioned was adamant that she'd had nothing. She also began complaining about excruciating stomach pains. A doctor was called and when he asked her about it she was unable to explain what the pain was like or where it was. Her answers were confused and incoherent and she became very distressed. She was given paracetamol to break her temperature (by making her sweat) and the doctor prescribed her Oramorph which is an oral morphine and extremely fast acting. She was also given a few other pain relief medications and thankfully the medication did its job; within half an hour the paracetamol had broken her temperature and she was sweating profusely, talking in coherent sentences and wondering why I was looking at her warily. Her pain had subsided and she was a million times better.

They believe that the pain is trapped wind which doesn't sound bad at all but can be excruciating – and for Mum that's exactly how it was. It can happen when you don't move very much – given that Mum spends 23.5 hours a day in bed it is little surprise that she has fallen foul of it. But it is so difficult to see her when she gets like this. I want to help her (at one point tonight she held my hand, weeping, and begged me to help her.) but there is nothing practical I can do. So tonight I did the only thing I could. I stroked her hand and promised I would help and that the doctor was on his way. This was enough for her and she drifted off again. She forgot it quickly but I can assure you I will not do the same. There have been many painful and distressing moments so far but this is one that will live in my memory. She is fragile and weak and in pain and I would do anything if it would help. But it won't. All I can do is what I did. And it seems so ridiculously inadequate.

But to end on a positive – she is not having negative reactions to the enhanced cells. Let's hope that continues.

xxx

# The End of the Road

It is with a broken heart and tear-blurred eyes that I type this. On Wednesday we were told by Mum's consultant that she is too weak for the transplant. Although the enhanced cells have fought some of the infections Mum is battling it has not beaten them all. There are too many. Also she is becoming immune to the antibiotics. So she will continue to get weaker.

So you can see, can't you, what I am trying desperately not to type? Mum has lost her fight. Without the transplant there is no hope of her beating this; and she will not be having a transplant. The road ahead is set. Although we can't say for certain when we will reach it, the destination is inevitable. And it will be sooner rather than later.

The hospital staff have been superb. She will continue to receive treatment until the end. There is talk of moving her to the Butterwick Hospice towards the end but we will see. Unfortunately she will not be coming home. She would need a bed and hoist installing downstairs, amongst other items, but even if we did that she would still need 24 hour nursing. And that is not possible. She will not be returning home.

We are broken; we are beaten. There are no words to describe the horror that we now face; the horror of life without her.

Your support at this time is appreciated beyond words.

xxx

# Palliative Care so Far

Since Wednesday it has been a bumpy road. Mum has, understandably, declined rapidly and it has been very difficult for us to watch. Although she has fought as hard as possible since July it would appear that last week's news has knocked all the fight out of her. And no one can blame her; what's the point in fighting if there is only one way this is all going to end? She seems to have accepted it with a weary finality that belies the fears she undoubtedly feels.

The hospital staff have continued to be amazing; they leave us be if she is having a difficult day but are there at any time we need them. Mum is often in a lot of pain and she is given a cocktail of medication to try and make her comfortable, including Morphine, Oramorph (a liquid morphine that she can swallow), Tamazepam, Tramadol and Paracetamol (although not all at the same time!!!)

She sleeps a lot of the time and this is good; she needs to rest and sleep so that the medication can take effect. Also, if she is sleeping she feels less pain. One of the most difficult things to see is the pain in her eyes. There are times that she is in tears and the only thing we can do is turn our heads so that she cannot see our tears threatening to spill down our cheeks.

Her days follow no real pattern; some days she sleeps the day away, others she barely closes her eyes. Her mood changes with the minutes: One minute she is lucid, then next confused and talking about events that happened a long time ago; one minute she is peaceful the next agitated and in pain; one minute calm the next wanting to get up and walk or sit in a chair (Which she cannot do because she is too weak.) The rollercoaster ride continues. As hard as it is for us, never knowing what to expect when we walk through her door, it is a joy and a blessing when she has 'better' moments. My fabulous Mum is obviously there, shining through and being cross with us for a variety of small transgressions. I find myself wishing fervently that these moments would become more frequent; unfortunately the opposite is the case. She fades a little more each day.

Earlier in the week they fitted a catheter because it was becoming increasingly difficult for her to get out of bed and she was too weak to support herself when sitting up or walking. Although this was a difficult decision for her to make we all feel it was the right one as it is one less thing for her to worry about.

So we continue to take things, at best, hour by hour; at times minute by minute.

As always, your thoughts and prayers are appreciated beyond words.

xxx

# Open Letter to Mum

Dear Mum,

Leaving you tonight was really difficult. After you fell asleep, the things I wanted to say to you began swirling round my head and it was all I could do not to wake you up and say them to you. I decided this would be better. The things I feel I want to say are difficult to articulate; mainly because they are mostly not about what has already *been* but about the future. About 'after', if you will.

You are my rock. One of, if not the, hardest thing about the last four months is that you are the one I turn to for strength. It has always been you. Any crisis that I have faced so far has been surmounted by listening to your advice (and lashings of tea or wine!), even when it seems I scoffed and scorned it. It is your hand I have sought when mine needed a reassuring squeeze; your lap I lay my head in when I need to weep; your smile that I seek through my tears. And now I find that I can't do any of those things I feel bereft. So many people have commented on how 'strong' I have been through this and I know that this strength comes from you. I am your daughter and much of who I am comes from you and the guidance you have always given; wanted or not! The strength I have shown comes from your teaching and the knowledge that you are proud of me, even with all the mistakes I have made.

I have lost count of the times in the last four months I have replayed memories from over the years. New York stands out – a whirlwind weekend of snow, ice, rip off cameras and memories that will last a lifetime. Holidays throughout the years, all of which have some sort of ridiculous event that none of us will ever forget (I'm thinking 'court of the klettering stick', broken bones, Daddo flippantly telling you that you were fine to ski down the mountain not knowing you had a torn cruciate ligament, lost perfume bottles, melted butter packs in shell-suit pockets, the list is endless). Will holidays ever be the same again? How on earth can I go away without knowing that at some point you will either do or say something which will become the focal point of any holiday story?

There are phrases that have become folk-lore thanks to you. The phrase 'damp crotch' will forever be met with laughs and grins and the recounting of the time you shouted to me and Tony from across a crowded plane en route to Portugal, "Ant, Tony, Lily has a bit of a DAMP CROTCH! Should I change her nappy?!" I will forever remember the cringing slink into the seat both Tony and I performed as we muttered, "Yes please!" and looked away hoping that we could suddenly become invisible. I never thought it possible but I now use this phrase at least once a week in order to raise a smile, either from me or from others familiar with the story. Or when in Scotland last year, out for a meal for Tony's birthday, you couldn't find the seatbelt in the back of the car, scrabbled around a bit then pronounced to us all, "Oh sorry, Tony, I'm just fingering your buttocks!" I am laughing just thinking about it. Mine and Dad's reaction was exactly the same: "Please stop!!!" T just laughed as I recall. He knew, as we all did, that it would become one of the best stories from the holiday; and it did.

Remember the pampering weekend with Holly and M2? Me screaming, "FRILLS?!?! FRILLS?!?! Just because I am pregnant does NOT mean I want to wear BLOODY FRILLS!!!" and you calmly, serenely, stating, "Pregnancy does seem to be making Antonia rather irritable. How are you two doing?"

But as I said earlier, the harder things to say are not about what has been, but about what has not. Next year is my big birthday. How on earth do I turn 30 without you? It is wrong and it scares me. We have thrown ideas around before now – a ceilidh for friends and family, an intimate dinner at a Michelin starred restaurant, one of your home cooked 'nothing fancy' seven course dinners. None of these will seem right without you. And yet it will happen.

My wedding day (if it happens) will be tinged with sadness because you will not be there. I have imagined us dress shopping and the arguments it will create. I can imagine your face and comments now: "Backless?!?! I don't think so…"; "Maybe if it was in a different material that wasn't so unflattering…"; "Why would you want lace?! It doesn't suit you"; "The colour does nothing for you"; "No. You look huge"; "You look stunning." (This would be the one that I hate and only tried on to shut you up.). So when (if) the day should come that I need to be in that situation, I will have to imagine you there, which we all know will be a pale comparison. It is wrong, Momma. It's just wrong.

There are hundreds of these moments that I see stretching ahead of me and it scares me. But worse, in a way, than those major events is the knowledge that we wasted so much time. We promised ourselves that we would go out for dinner once a month. We never did. On the rare occasion we went out we loved it. Why didn't we do it more? I wish, more than anything, that we had. As someone special said to me recently, "Often life gets in the way." And it did. It so did. And I wish more than anything that it hadn't. We promised ourselves weekends away, pampering sessions, shopping trips, dancing lessons, gym sessions, coffee…why, instead of promising them did we not just do them?

You are the best grandma to my girls. I watched you playing with Lily and was grateful that she had such an amazing and strong woman as a role model. She was lucky that you and Dad looked after her, played with her, taught her. Alba didn't have as long but the smile she gets on her face when she sees you, even your picture, demonstrates the impact you have had on her short life. Thanks to you Lily can ride a bike, 'play softly' on the piano(!), bake, paint, write her name…again the list is endless. Now I will have to be twice the mum to make up for you not being there. I promise to try, Momma, is that enough?

I wish that I had let you teach me how to cook. And that I had got your lasagne recipe. I wish I had raided your wardrobe and pinched things while you were still able to shout at me because you wanted to wear it and I had not returned it. I wish I had learned how to sew so that when Big Bear needs surgery, Lily won't look at me in disgust when I do a botched job and declare, "I should have given it to Grandma, Mummy. She'd have done a good job." I wish I had told you every day how much I love you and how proud I am of you and how proud I am to be your and Dad's daughter. I wish, I wish I wish…

There's more, but you get the gist. More would be too much. Too much for me to bear, too much for you to read, too much for Dad, too much…just too much.

So, I hear you thinking, what is the point of this, Antonia? What is the point of this self-indulgent letter? Is it just to make you feel better and everyone else feel worse? OR was there something else? Well here it is, Momma. Here is what I wanted to say: Thank you. Thank you for the last 29 years. And thank you for the future I have ahead of me. You have prepared me for it, you have laid the pathway and shown me the right way from the wrong. You have held my hand, guided me, corrected me, berated me, but most of all, MOST OF ALL, you have loved me, uncompromisingly, uncomplicatedly and unconditionally.

I love you, Momma. I will always love you.

Goodnight, God bless. Sweet dreams.

I love you to the moon and back.

xxx

# Good Night

Mum lost her fight on Sunday, 1 December.
Goodnight Mum.
I love you to the moon and back.

    xxx

# Funeral

Mum's funeral will be held at St. Mary's Church, Longnewton on Wednesday, 11 December at 12.45. More details to follow.

xxx

# Stumbling Through

And so we stumble through the minutes, hours and days. We swing from 'fine' to wretched in one fell swoop. We are numb; we are devastated; we are. And she is not. And at the moment it hasn't sunk in, it has not hit us. We let down our guard and it hits. And we cry. But then we pick ourselves up and continue. Because what else can we do? There are things to do, people to call, arrangements to be made.

But what will happen when that stops? When there are no phone calls, when there is no one left to be told, when the arrangements are not only made but have come to fruition; what then? I don't know. All I know is that I miss her; desperately, horribly, fruitlessly. She is no longer here and I cannot talk directly to her, hug her directly, laugh directly with her. But I will do all those things indirectly. I still speak to her and so I should – Mum spoke to Grandma frequently even though she knew that she couldn't answer. I feel her arms around me – and I will never stop because her hugs were copious and wonderful and I was lucky to have so many of them. I will laugh (eventually) and think of her – for she gave me so many reasons to laugh.

She was my mum and she was amazing. And (as two special people have pointed out to me in recent days) you all knew her but she was my mum. And I will be eternally grateful for that. Because, when it comes down to it, who could ask for a more wonderful mother and guide? No one.

I will continue to write because it helps. I may not be able to articulate a lot of what I am feeling but with my fingers hovering over the keyboard somehow it all flows out. And (as I try to teach my pupils to do) I edit as I go along, I write, and then delete, and then rewrite. And even though it is not always perfect it makes sense. To me anyway. And when it doesn't make complete sense, when it seems a little confused or it doesn't quite 'flow' (or I feel too many sentences begin with the word 'and'), I remind myself that not so very long ago, in a moment of lucidity, my mum told me how proud she was of my writing. And for me, that is enough. For now at any rate.

xxx

# Vacant

A difficult day today. Lots of things to do, lots of people to speak to, lots of words said; none of them remembered. I find I cannot retain things just now. A conversation had five minutes ago will either be forgotten or recalled as though it happened a week ago. I bumble around consulting a list of things which need to be done and somehow at the end of the day they are done. Then I write a new list – a list of things to be done tomorrow. It is the only way I currently see of getting through the long hours that stretch ahead of me. So the funeral is now arranged.

St Mary's Church, Wednesday, 11 December, 12.45.

The service is planned, the hymns chosen, the people involved know, the Centre is booked for afterwards, the caterers called, the crematorium booked for close family.

Dad and I support each other; and Tony is amazing. No pressure to do anything, just constant, gentle support for each new challenge we face. Our ongoing task is tackling Dad's house. It is showing the strain of the last five months almost as much as we are. It feels in disarray, slightly neglected, forlorn. Each day we tackle a new room, putting away, tidying, shuffling piles into a different room. We throw away nothing for we are not ready but we are trying to hide the evidence. Just putting things in the correct cupboard so they are less 'in your face' is a help: We know what is behind the cupboard door but at least we don't have to see it.

Each day I drag myself out of bed and into the shower. The face I see in the mirror is undoubtedly mine yet sometimes I fail to recognise me. My eyes are dead; vacant. I can cry, laugh, shout, snap, wail and a whole host of other things but there is something which has gone. Some part of me that is missing. I presume it is with Mum. And to me this is acceptable at the moment. It feels completely understandable. I just hope that one day, in the future (dim and distant though it may be) someone looks into my eyes and smiles and says, "Hi. You're back." And then I will know that, just maybe, I am starting to come through this.

xxx

# There's a Tree in My Living Room

There is a fully decorated Christmas tree in my living room. Which can only mean one thing; despite this monumental, devastating and life-changing event, the world keeps on turning. That's a hard lesson to learn. As I sleepwalk through the hours, everyone else is bobbing along nicely. Most people try to hide this from me. Some people are too open about it. But the best people (or friends as I call them) strike the right balance between listening to me ramble and distracting me with their stories. For this I will be eternally grateful.

We had to tell Lily. I didn't for a while; I couldn't. It made it all so…real. She is devastated. But in the way children have, she will pick herself up and continue. Her first thought was for Grandy. Her tear-stained face was stricken with panic as she asked the most important question, "But who will live with Grandy? Who will look after him?" The reply was so obvious I almost, *almost*, managed a smile as I answered, "We will." For we will. We will all look after each other. We have all been knifed by this and so we will all get through it together. And I know that sounds really glib and cliché but it is because it is true. Each day I spend time with my dad; he'll get sick of me soon. We make a list of things that we have to do and then we do it. Then we make a mental list of what we have to do tomorrow. And then…well you get the drift. I don't know what will happen when the inevitable day comes; the day when we have nothing that needs to be done. Perhaps we will sit in silence, staring at each other and the four walls. Or perhaps we will begin to carefully, feebly, cautiously put our lives back together and piece by little piece, step by little step, work out how we go about living again.

But we couldn't explain all that to Lily, not properly. So we did our best, we answered every question she threw at us, we read an AMAZING book *Water Bugs and Dragonflies* and we tried to soothe her as she wept. And we tried diversion tactics. Like choosing a Christmas tree; then decorating it; writing Christmas cards; then posting them. And so far it seems to have worked. She asks the most random questions at the most inopportune times. But we try our best to answer them. What else can we do? She is too young to understand terms like 'grief' and to understand that everyone is just as sad as she is. And I don't want her to understand yet, I want her to continue as she is; because it seems so healthy. She is getting on, crying when she needs to, laughing when she needs to, asking the questions, but most importantly she is remembering her grandma for the wonderful, fun loving, inspirational person she was. And, to me, that seems just right.

xxx

# Eulogy

The funeral was on Wednesday. This is the Eulogy. It was only a small part of the service, however. Mum chose the hymns before she died so we had: I stand alone in the presence of Jesus the Nazarene; How deep the father's love for us; The Lord's my shepherd I'll not want (the new version); How great thou art. The reading was John 21. 4-17. There was a beautiful Address by John, our vicar (and friend), Church Tributes, and prayers led by members of the church. It was a beautiful and fitting tribute to my amazing mother.

The eulogy was written by Dad and I; the writing of it was mixed with tears and smiles. The more we wrote, the more we remembered, the more we smiled, the more we laughed, the more we cried. As I wrote I realised that I couldn't include anything about my dad, me, my children, Tony, my sisters and so on. Because it was too flipping hard. It was too personal. I'm not ready to share that yet. But with this came the realisation that although we originally wrote it for someone else to read (we both thought it would be difficult for us to read aloud) as I read it back I realised that what shone through the writing, alongside how bloody amazing my mum was, was me. It was my voice that came through, my thoughts, my memories, and (I hope) my love for my mum. Ando so there was only one option: I had to read it. It was one of the hardest things I have ever done. To stand next to her coffin and read this out; would she be proud or would she be peeved that I included the stories I did? Would she think I did well or criticise how fast I read it? (I know which I think.) But I did it. I got through it. I did it for Mum and I am proud. I think she would have been.

So here it is, for anyone who missed it, or anyone who wants to read it again. The family Eulogy:

My mum, Dee, was born on 23 August 1949. She was the first born child of Jim and Sonia and was to become the eldest of four sisters; a role that she felt challenged her at times beyond her capabilities. From learning to cook in order to feed hungry sisters after school snacks, to replacing smashed mixing bowls before her mum got home and realised it was broken, her early life was filled with responsibility but also fun. She would often recount tales about her father coming home from work and throwing all the cushions off the sofa to make 'islands' for them all to jump on. Then, having glimpsed Sonia getting off the bus from work, frantically sweeping everything up and back into its place.

From the start she and her sisters shared a bond that was fiercely close and protective. And whilst they were happy to tell on each other they would turn on anyone who dared to hurt their family in any way. This protectiveness would appear in every relationship and friendship that she experienced.

Dee loved education and believed it to be the only means to equality. However, it was not always plain sailing for her. Her first day of school left her distraught after she was told by the dinner lady 'you can go'. She took this to mean she could go home, rather than out to play, and so was bewildered when she arrived on her doorstep to be met by a furious Sonia who promptly marched her back to school. Despite these inauspicious beginnings she grew to love education and dedicated her working life to the improvement of it.

She enjoyed school and was proud to be awarded the title of Deputy Head girl at Grangefield Grammar School. From there she went on to Wall Hall Training College and trained to be a teacher. Her first teaching job was at Billingham Campus, followed by Northfield where her flair for Drama came into its own. The school plays became a byword for quality and few who witnessed them will ever forget *Antigone, Charlie and the Chocolate Factory, The*

*Government Inspector* and in particular *Oh What a Lovely War* with her and Ian's skit becoming the talk of the cast after party. She was then appointed as, first Head of English, then Deputy Head at Nunthorpe School in Middlesbrough. Under the guidance of John Rowling she flourished, as did the school. This must also be attributed in part to her heated arguments with Steven Prandle, the other deputy. These arguments were without malice but came from deep convictions and principles.

From there, she progressed to Head of Brakenhoe school. It was not an easy area to work in and Dee faced many challenges; but she always put the pupils and their families first. She believed that every child has the right to a good education and that sentiment was the driving force behind many of her decisions.

Eventually, she decided that it was time to move on and she took on the role of Project Manager of the EAZ (Education Action Zone) in Middlesbrough; a government initiative focussed on improving the quality of education in deprived areas. Dee's passion for the arts shone through in this role as one of her priorities became introducing children to a world of music, art, drama and performance that was hitherto unknown to them. Her journey through the world of work then took her to Project Manager of TEEP, working for The Sainsbury Family Trust. Her work was pioneering in education and with her help thousands of classroom teachers throughout the UK were able to improve their day-to-day practice, and thereby improve the education of thousands of pupils.

This role took her far and wide and her influence spread not just throughout the UK but also to Australia, America, Cyprus and Dubai. She not only made work colleagues but acquired close friends along the way.

Guiding Dee throughout her life was her deep faith. She became an active member of the Church holding many roles and juggling many commitments; always with a smile and a want to help, support and spread the good word. Her style shone through especially in her Preaching. Many of the congregation looked forward to the services when her unique style of delivery would brighten the greyest Sunday morning. PCC, MDT, Little Ted, leading services, preaching, prayers, GodZone, being a very vocal member of the choral group, homegroup, Deputy Chair of governors at St. Mary's Primary School: the list goes on. Her influence was enormous. But with this enormous influence came an even greater humility. And it is for that more than anything that she will be remembered and missed within the church.

The one place Dee failed miserably was on the sports field. Never a holiday passed without some mishap, generally related to her falling, tripping, stumbling or generally breaking something, somehow, in the most ridiculous ways. She once managed to break her toe climbing out of the bath. Few however will forget THE skiing story. The one where Dee fell over, and screamed in agony only to be met with Ian's brusque response of "You'll be fine, just rest there at the bottom of this lift. Ant and I will just go and do this Black Run then we'll all ski down together". How was he to know she'd torn her cruciate ligament? Or the time she fell over and complained her ribs were sore; it turns out she'd cracked two. No one could work out how until she sheepishly admitted that she'd had her purse, which was full to the brim with coins, stuffed inside her ski suit and had fallen on it which was probably what had cracked her ribs. But she was not one to let her lack of sporting prowess deter her and would gamely give it a go despite knowing it would probably not end well.

Despite her failures in the world of sport, she surpassed herself with her cooking skills. She was never happier than when in the kitchen cooking a simple 'Nothing fancy' meal (which usually consisted of around seven courses!). But it was 'nothing fancy'. Her lasagne is legendary; her panna cotta, one tasted, is never to be forgotten. And that Italian flair was not only to be found in her food. Her fiery temper would flare up and die away quickly. It is, apparently, a family trait, and many have been surprised at the heat with which Mum and I would argue in the kitchen (where else?). However if anyone tried to intervene the response would chorus from us both, in stereo, "Oh leave us alone! We enjoy it!" before resuming our argument.

A more calming interest of hers was needlecraft. Her quilts decorate many houses and were made and given with such love that the missed stitches or slight imperfections serve as a fond reminder that even though things weren't always perfect, it doesn't matter because they were done with love. It is heart wrenching that she finished her sewing room in June this year, and despite looking forward to using it and creating masterpieces in it, she never got to use it.

She touched and influenced for good so many lives that it is at times inconceivable that she is no longer here. She was an amazing, wonderful, inspirational force; and although she is gone her influence is not. And her spirit lives on in us all.

# Step by Little Step

Since the funeral, it seems like a lot has happened, yet not a lot at the same time. Each day poses challenges old and new. The first one of each day is forcing myself out of bed. Once that is accomplished I feel I am on a bit of a roll and somehow manage to get through the rest of the day. Christmas is a bit of a blur; the girls had a good day and we saw family. Boxing Day saw us out for a walk on the beach followed by dinner at my sister's. It was all very different from normal but in this instance different was good. There was no parody of Christmas' past; no pretending that it was all fine and as it should be but with a gaping hole where Mum should have been. Different felt, if not right, then better than the alternative. I was very lucky to have such wonderful family and friends around me to keep me going.

People repeatedly told me that the girls would help me get through it, and in some respects they have. However bad I am feeling they still need their mum; clothes still need washing; cupboards still need stocking; Santa still had to visit. In other ways it made it a little harder. Some days all I desperately wanted to do was to pull the covers over my head and stay in my 'nest' until it felt safe to come out. I have had very little time by myself and I felt this keenly a few weeks ago. I'd had a little time to myself and broke down. I wept for an hour, wrote a letter to Mum and went to bed. It was cathartic. It helped.

Mainly I try not to think too much. About anything. Instead I focus on 'chunking' the day up and achieving one small step at a time. That way I get through the day with the added bonus of being exhausted each evening and guaranteeing some sleep. (Alba has other ideas and has decided to stop sleeping on a night but that is another story entirely.)

I have been referred for bereavement counselling which, I think, is a positive step. During my initial assessment, the girl/woman asked me what I hoped to achieve by having counselling. For a moment I was silent; I wasn't expecting that question and so didn't have an answer prepared. When it did arrive my answer surprised me. I told her I wasn't expecting to 'achieve' anything: I just wanted the opportunity to talk through what I am (or am not) feeling in the hope of making some sense of it. I want to understand how I feel about everything that has happened and how I feel about what is to come. Apparently, this was the right answer and I am 'the perfect candidate for the service'. This was strangely comforting. I just hope that I feel better after the sessions.

Life rolls on and time keeps ticking. One day it may feel like it's back to its normal speed.

xxx

# Sorting Through

In the past few days there have been some really low points. The lowest being when Dad and I started the mammoth task of sorting through Mum's belongings.

Last week I brought home her jewellery; Mum had loads of items, most of them costume but some of them more expensive. The problem was that she treated them all the same regardless of value. Which means that I brought home five boxes, all crammed, full to the brim, with an assortment of earrings, bracelets, necklaces and broaches. It took me three hours to sort them out into 'categories' and then a further four hours for my friend to help me identify the more valuable items. So seven hours spent handling things that were precious to my mum, most of which evoked memories of when I was little: sitting on her bed watching her get ready; trying on her clip on earrings and feeling very grown up; twisting her long rope necklaces around my wrist as I snuggled sleepily in her lap...the memories were endless. And unimaginably painful. But with the sadness was pleasure; pleasure that I was holding something that was indefatigably 'mum'. She was never seen without some item of jewellery and holding each piece, letting the cool metal slip through my fingers, made me smile as much as it made me weep. I am more grateful than I can express that I will have these tangible memories of her.

Sorting the jewellery led quite obviously to sorting through her clothes. Dad and I started this yesterday. The biggest question was what to do with them. A charity shop is the obvious answer but which one? We haven't decided yet but there are wardrobes full of clothes. Mum loved clothes as much as she loved jewellery. And stored them in a similar manner. So today I went through two wardrobes looking for suits that I may be able to wear. (This is the perfect place to point out that my mum had superb taste and loved brands such as Hobbs, L.K. Bennett, Wallis etc.) Although there is an obvious age difference between Mum and me and many of her clothes are, not to put too fine a point on it, far too old for me, she also favoured timeless classics, especially when it came to suits and work wear. And luckily for me we were similar sizes. So today my search began.

Many people tell you how you have to 'wait until you are ready' and that 'it gets easier' and so on. What they don't tell you is that when you open a wardrobe door that has been closed for five months, the smell that hits you is impregnated with sadness, loss and nostalgia. I cried buckets today. Every item of clothing smelled of Mum. 90% had special memories attached. The other 10% was almost worse because they still had labels on; they were filled with promises of the future which are never going to be fulfilled: evening dresses to be worn on the next cruise Mum and Dad were to take; shirts that were delivered the week before she went into hospital; jeans that were worn once while on holiday and she loved but never got the chance to wear again. At times I found it hard to swallow past the burning lump in my throat. I didn't want to be there, going through her things, without her there with me. I wanted her to be sitting on the bed, as she always did, commenting (often harshly) on the clothes I was trying on. And though Dad tried, we both knew it wasn't quite right; just as life isn't right without her. Tomorrow we make a start on her shoes. We are saving the bigger things until we feel stronger.

I have thought of Mum constantly since the funeral, adjusting and adapting to life without her. But yesterday and today made her absence more real. Although we have 'thrown out' nothing, the process has started which means that she irrefutably is not coming back. We finally took down the condolence cards yesterday and Dad commented, 'It seems empty without them.' We both cried because we knew that what we really felt was that it seems empty without Mum.

Nothing seems right, our world seems a little empty, the sun doesn't shine as brightly (or at all some days), colours have lost their vibrancy, sounds are muted; and cutting through it all is the sharp searing pain of loss. It hasn't faded or dimmed or dulled or gone anywhere.

One day, maybe, but not yet.

xxx

# I Stand Amazed...

This weekend was difficult. It was the 'big family get together'; which basically involves me, T, our two girls, my older sister, brother-in law and their two boys, our middle sister and middle brother-in-law, and Dad. And that's why it was so difficult. Because the end of that sentence should read 'and Mum and Dad'. What usually happens is that we all descend on Mum and Dad's house sometime between Christmas and New Year, Mum cooks a fabulous 'nothing fancy' meal, we drink good wine (Dad's) and play the best game in the world 'Tell Me') amidst shrieks of '1984!', 'Hoover!', 'Bean bag slippers!' and 'Tyrannosaurus Rex!' (none of which will mean anything to you unless you have played the game 'Tell Me' whilst slightly tipsy after a fabulous bottle or three of red wine) and raucous laughter. But this year was different of course.

For a start, none of us cooked. It would have felt so wrong. No one could (can) cook better than Mum, so why would we try? It would simply highlight the fact that she was not there. So instead we ordered takeaway (Chinese, if you're interested.). It was fine. We drank – but not as much as usual because it was a slightly subdued evening. Although we all tried really hard, there was no escaping the fact that at some point in the evening every single one of us carried something into the kitchen and fully expected to see her standing, pinny on, washing up, or taking something delicious out of the oven, or bending over the dishwasher, or just leaning against the counter with a glass of wine in her hands. And at that moment when she realised she wasn't there, every single one of us caught our breath and felt that knife twist deep in our chest.

We pushed through it of course. Few will quickly forget the sight of Viv, Lily and I playing twister on the smallest mat ever seen, while the boys looked on, slightly bemused expressions creasing their brows. The piano was played for a bit, although that was painful to hear because as beautifully as Kevin played, it was Mum who always had to begin the begging for him to play for us all. And so when he did it without prompting there was a tear in my eye – and I wasn't alone. The evening was, in all, delightful. We all thoroughly enjoyed ourselves, even if I did argue with both brother-in-laws. They know me well enough now to know that I say things mostly to get a rise out of them and that there is no malice in anything I say (and if they don't they flipping well should!). I know you can't speak for other people but I think Dad enjoyed himself. And when we realised how late it was (bad parents all round having our children out so late) although we felt a bit guilty, we also revelled in the fact that it was only because we had been enjoying ourselves so much.

But oh how I missed her. Oh how I wish she was there. Tony and I talked after we'd put the girls to bed, about how hard it was. And I think for him it was especially hard – it was the first time that he has been in a situation where her presence lingers and her absence is tangible. And while I wanted to comfort him I also couldn't help but say 'That's how I feel, every second, every minute of every day.' And then I hugged him. Because we all loved her. We all miss her terribly. And we all deal with it in our own ways. I stay quiet and pour it out to this blog when I need to. Tony channels it into looking after me and the girls. Dad – Dad is just Dad. We do our best to support each other, to reach out to each other, but every now and again, just as we think we are standing a little but taller, something comes and blasts us and we are back on our knees.

Like the service at church last Sunday. All was going fine until the last hymn appeared on the screen and without warning we found ourselves rising to sing 'I stand amazed at the presence of Jesus the Nazarene.' And I couldn't. I managed to choke out the first two lines before my throat closed up and I cried and cried. Because that was Mum's hymn; and all I could see as I stared at the screen was her, standing at the front, arms swinging, head up high, voice soaring forth, loving life, loving her God, and loving every one who stood in front of her. So I end this post with a verse that sums up my feelings for her. For 'He' substitute 'she', for 'saviour' substitute 'mother' and you will see just a fraction of how wonderful my mother was and why I miss her so very very much. For you, Mum.

*'For me it was in the garden,*
*He said not my will but thine.*
*He had no tears for his own sin,*
*but sweat drops of blood for mine.*
*How marvellous, how wonderful,*
*And my soul shall ever be.*
*How marvellous, how wonderful,*
*Is my saviours love for me.'*

xxx

# A Short Story

Once upon a time (11am this morning), a small group of people gathered in a church yard. They formed a circle around a small, square, freshly dug hole. Amongst the group were a vicar, a widower, a young mother and two sets of sisters. On a morning which was surreal in its tranquillity and sunlight, they gathered to say a final farewell to a woman whose loss has not even begun to make itself truly felt. Words were said, prayers offered, tears shed; and throughout it all a sense of calm prevailed. The sun shone and the birds sang and the traffic quietened and it was beautiful.

The placement of the hole had been chosen by the woman they were all there to honour. It is next to her neighbour and as close as possible to the church. Both these details were important to her. As the small group stood and watched the casket lowered into the hole they cried. All eight of them. Because this ending, this beautiful, calm and quiet ceremony, was perfectly in keeping with what she had wanted. Her nearest and dearest were there to say a final farewell.

In time a stone will be placed, it will be simple but elegant – just like her. And it will mark the place where she has been laid to rest. It will be visited frequently, by family and friends alike. It will stand as a testament to the love we had for her, and the love we received from her. It will be there to remind us that although she may not be with us in person, her influence will always be with us.

That woman was my mother and I will love her unto eternity.

# Post Script
## One Year Later
## Here's What I Know
## 1 December 2014

Here's what I know: Grief doesn't magically go away. You can hate yourself for smiling. Sometimes you forget and then it all comes crashing back. Children have a knack of twisting a knife in your heart with a wrongly timed question and absolutely no malice meant. I've grown up. I will never not miss her. I will always love her.

A year ago today, my life changed irrevocably. The past year has been a myriad of emotions and experiences. Not a day goes by when I do not feel, remember and grieve the loss of such a fabulous woman. The woman who made me who I am; the woman who showed me who I want to be; the woman who gave me the belief that I can be who I want and that that will be fabulous; the woman I look up to more than anyone else; the woman I love. She taught me so much and this time last year I was wondering who would teach me now she is gone. I did not expect the answer I have discovered; she has taught me even though she is no longer here.

Every day (if not every hour, minute, second) I find myself asking her advice. I wonder what she would do, what she would say, what she would think. And every time I find my answer. Not by 'a voice' in my head, not by 'signs', but by the principles she taught me over the years and the grounding she gave me. She paved the way for me to grow up. She gave me the basics with which to go on without her.

She loved me and let me know it and because of that I have not curled up and withdrawn from the world (or at least, not very often) but have got up, got dressed and faced the world.

I wish that she was here to see that I have grown up. I wish that she could see my daughters grow up. I wish that she was coming here on Christmas Day with the rest of the family. But that cannot happen. However, because of her, because of the role model she was, I know that she was confident that this would all happen. She knew that I would step up, that I would be a good mum, that one day I would host Christmas and make it a different day to the one we used to have but one that is just as special for my girls and family. She knew all this because she is the one who taught me how.

There are a million moments when I have wanted to speak to her. To shout at her. To rant to her. To put my arms around her and hug her, to kiss her on the cheek, to tell her I love her one last time. The first three of these I do, sometimes out loud, sometimes in my head, sometimes on paper in letters which will never be sent but always kept. But the last three I can't. And that's hard. But not as hard as realising that I can't quite remember the touch of her hand on my forehead. Or her lips brushing my cheek. Or the exact lilt of her laugh. I am lucky enough to have videos and photos but they can't convey her touch. They reignite my memory of her but they can't recreate the moment and that is what, in the long, dark, difficult days, I miss more than anything. I long for her arms to steal around me and squeeze me gently; on a lucky night she appears in my dreams and does just that. I wake with the weight of her arms around me only to find them fading with the sunlight which streams through the window. It hurts almost as much as not being able to quite remember.

Some mornings I wake with her name on my lips and my tears on my pillow and know I have been dreaming of her. Those mornings I feel blessed.

It is in church that I often weep because I can almost see her, arms swinging as she sang, a smirk twitching her lips as we shared a look, a private joke, unspoken but understood by just a tweak of an eyebrow. It is hard to go there each Sunday and feel her memory surrounding me; but it is a good pain. It is a pain that feels healing as opposed to destructive. I *want* to remember her; I never want to forget.

Christingle was hard for last year it fell on the 1st of December so she and it will be forever linked in my mind. Someone once said she was the light of the Church; she was the light of my life. She was what guided me, she was my means of navigation in difficult times, she was what I reached for when things were good and bad, she was comfort, she was safe, she was love. She was everything. We all miss her but we are slowly, carefully, cautiously rebuilding our lives. One tiny, tinchy, smidgeon at a time.

One year has passed; many more stretch ahead. Thank you, Mum, for giving me the strength to face whatever they may bring.

xxx